MEDICAL REVOLUTION IN FRANCE
1789-1796

MEDICAL REVOLUTION IN FRANCE 1789-1796

DAVID M. VESS

A Florida State University Book
University Presses of Florida
Gainesville

Library of Congress Cataloging in Publication Data

Vess, David M
    Medical revolution in France, 1789–1796.

    "A Florida State University book."
    Bibliography: p.
    1. Medicine–France–History. 2. France–
History–Revolution, 1789-1799–Medical and sanitary
affairs. I. Title. [DNLM: 1. History of medicine,
18th century–France. 2. Military medicine–
History–France. WZ70 GF7 V5m]
R504.V47   610'.944   74-14916
ISBN 0-8130-0439-X

CONTENTS

PREFACE

It is a special pleasure to record here that Professor John Fraser Ramsey of the University of Alabama suggested this study. His painstaking guidance and meticulous scholarship have been of great benefit to the manuscript. His friendship and unfailing confidence in me have been important in its fruition. For patient, careful reading and many helpful suggestions, I am also indebted to Professor Donald D. Horward of the Florida State University and to Professor Bernerd C. Weber and the late Professor Wilburt S. Brown of the University of Alabama. However, I assume full responsibility and beg indulgence for any omissions or inaccuracies that the reader may find.

The opportunity to deal definitively with this subject was provided by a sabbatical leave and a research grant afforded me by Samford University. I am deeply grateful for both, especially for Samford University Research Grant No. 21, which made possible a period of intensive research in the archival collections in Paris.

Deep appreciation is extended to General Baylon, head of the French Military Medical Service and Director of the Army's Medical School and Teaching Hospital in Paris, who granted broad permission for the use of the Central Library and Historical Archives of the Medical Service. Equally cordial and helpful was M. E. Vialard, Curator of the Musée Val-de-Grâce, who gave every possible assistance and encouragement. Access to the Archives of the Historical Service of the Army at Vincennes was provided through the courtesy of General Cantarel, Chief of Staff for the Army Ground Forces, General of Division Fournier, and Colonel Hurbin of the Army Historical Service. Other resources which were graciously made available to me were the Archives Nationales, the Bibliothèque Nationale, and the Bibliothèque de la Faculté de Médecine in Paris.

I wish to acknowledge with gratitude other libraries which have so generously aided my research. The Harwell G. Davis Library at Samford

University accorded me every help. Miss Helen Stamps, a superb reference librarian, performed some miracles in my behalf. In addition to the resources of the Main Library and the Science Library of the University of Alabama at Tuscaloosa, of indispensable assistance were the University of Alabama Medical Center Library in Birmingham and Mrs. Hilda G. Harris, the reference librarian. Located in the Medical Center also is the Lawrence Reynolds Historical Library where I was given access to a great number of rare sources and received hospitable and invaluable assistance from Mrs. Martha Lou Thomas, the rare book librarian. In addition, access to specific materials has left me indebted to the following: the Library of Congress; the National Library of Medicine and the Edward Rhodes Stitt Library at Bethesda, Maryland; Maxwell Air Force Base Library; the Library of the College of Physicians at Philadelphia; the Downstate Medical Center Library of the State University of New York at Brooklyn; the University of Wisconsin Medical Library; the J. Hillis Miller Health Center Library of the University of Florida; and the libraries of Johns Hopkins University, the State University of Iowa, the University of Iowa, the University of Kentucky, Harvard University, the University of North Carolina, and the Florida State University.

A personal expression of appreciation is due to my wife, Jean, who worked that I might study and who made large contributions of typing and proofreading as well as of love, encouragement, and patience. Our son John (now 21) preserved through seven years a good-natured and considerate spirit. This brief mention is scant reward for their sacrifices but I am very thankful for them.

Because this study has been in press for over 3 years, I would like to call attention to several recent works. While these studies in no way affect my thesis or conclusions, they are very valuable for details which might have enhanced several areas of this work. Students of this period will not want to overlook J. Gilchrist and W. J. Murray, *The Press in the French Revolution* (N.Y.: St. Martin's Press, 1971); Roger Hahn, *The Anatomy of a Scientific Institution: The Paris Academy of Sciences, 1666–1803* (Berkeley: University of California Press, 1971); Pierre Huard, *Sciences, Médecine, Pharmacie de la Révolution à l'Empire, 1789–1815* (Paris: R. Dacosta, 1970); and Alison Patrick, *The Men of the First French Republic* (Baltimore: Johns Hopkins Press, 1972).

David M. Vess

INTRODUCTION

Accustomed to numbered streets and avenues, an American in Paris is struck immediately by the great names of the French past that designate her streets, boulevards, and even subway stops. A student of the Revolution feels strangely at home on the boulevards Davout, Jourdan, Ney, Kellermann, Macdonald, Masséna, Murat, and Soult because he can quickly conjure up a vision of the brilliant marshals and the glittering legions of the armies of Napoleon I. Equally familiar are the place-names commemorating the political and literary giants of that era. But perhaps most surprisingly pleasant is the discovery of streets named for Bichat, Brillat-Savarin, Hallé, and Parmentier and subway stations memorializing Corvisart and Daubenton.

For one who has an interest in the history of French medicine, there is great satisfaction in an afternoon stroll on the Left Bank east from Napoleon's tomb at the Invalides, past the spires of St. Clotilde, down the Boulevard Saint Germain to the Ancienne Faculté de Médecine of the Rue des Saints Pères, past the School of Medicine to the Rue Saint Jacques, turning south past the Sorbonne, and on down to the Val-de-Grâce. Or one may head south from the Invalides past the Hospital Laënnec, the Children's Hospital, and the Necker, to the Pasteur Institute and beyond to the Hospital Broussais, then turn east to the Hospital Cochin, the Pitié, and the Salpêtrière, past the Jardin des Plantes, and then back to the Hôtel-Dieu on the Ile de la Cité. Seeing the great medical landmarks of the French past is a sufficient stimulation to the historian to attempt to recapture for others something of the excitement and significance of the turbulent revolutionary era in which French medicine was thrust into the modern world.

Any consideration of the medical revolution that was rooted in the French Revolution requires, first of all, a survey of the state of French medicine prior to 1789. The medical world of the eighteenth century was steeped in tradition and Hippocratic dogma and dominated by "library" or folklore medicine. The prevalence of a whole gamut of "philosophies" of medicine made its practice highly individualistic, with incredible variations of approaches and effectiveness among physicians and surgeons, whether urban or rural. The schemes for training medical men ranged from brief apprenticeships to a highly formal and rigidly restricted program of studies, while the profession was so loosely safeguarded that many amateurs simply proclaimed themselves "physicians" and commenced medical practice. The prerevolutionary scene also encompassed a complex network of medical organizations, institutions, and facilities. Civilian and military, public and private, these involved support from the State, the Church, private philanthrophy, and, usually, from all three combined in some way. The whole structure of medicine rested upon centuries past; on the eve of the Revolution, it had changed very little since the Middle Ages.

The initial impact of the Revolution was profoundly destructive of the old medicine and its institutions. To many Frenchmen, medicine epitomized the worst ills of the Old Regime: favoritism, monopoly, ineffectiveness, neglect, and ignorance. Justified by the revolutionaries as an essential part of the task of eradicating all vestiges of the society that they considered totally corrupt and without any redeeming quality, their sweeping decrees paralyzed or abolished medical organizations, hospitals, and medical schools, both civilian and military. The ideology of equality was extended to cover the medical profession; not only did surgeons and pharmacists become the equals of physicians but patients became the equals of their doctors. While this concept ultimately made talent the principal criterion for a successful career in medicine and surgery, it produced immediate chaos by licensing for medical practice a host of amateurs, quacks, and anyone else willing to pay the small fee. French medicine could scarcely have been dealt a more demoralizing and shattering blow.

Paralleling these developments were the shifting thought patterns of the revolutionaries during the 1790s. Some of them, rabidly anti-intellectual, dismissed medicine as a "worthless art." Some saw the profession as a threat to the principle of equality and insisted that anyone could practice so simple a craft; others extolled the healing qualities of Nature and felt that a proper medical education consisted primarily of developing the qualities of patriotism, virtue, and morality. The survival of the medical profession seemed to depend upon those who recognized the Republic's need for competent physicians and surgeons. Significant in this struggle was the role of many persons in the legislative assemblies, including many doctor-politicians, who attempted to structure a new concept of public responsibility for medical care and social assistance. Because they were convinced of the direct relationship between inadequate medical care and the indigence and misery of the people, a new public policy on health care finally emerged. Although these men could scarcely foresee it, this new national concern for the health of the people provided a fertile seedbed in which the new medicine could flourish.

Not until 1792, when the French republic went to war with Austria and Prussia, was there a slowing of the destructive thrust of the Revolution. A growing concern for effective health care for the citizen volunteers of the armies of 1792 reawakened an appreciation for the role of medicine and surgery in wartime. Therefore, when hostilities began, French military medicine assumed a significant role in the process of reconstructing the medical profession. This was a task fully as difficult as the reconstitution of the government or the reorganization of the economy, and it was complicated by the wartime emergency. Having no authorized organization, lacking funds, and hampered by hundreds of newly licensed amateurs, the military medical service during 1792 had to improvise an organization and the means of caring for the sick and wounded of the Revolution's mass armies.

Surgery, separated from medicine for centuries, had been steadily approximating medicine during the eighteenth century because the two found in pathological anatomy and experimental physiology a common ground. Clinicism, hospital reform, and medicine's steady absorption of the accessory sciences and technology provided the backdrop for a new approach to medicine. Perhaps best labeled by Ackernecht as "hospital medicine,"[1] it was nourished in the new type of hospital, both civilian and military, that had to be created during the 1790s to care for the hordes of sick and wounded. In this institution could be developed three essential supports of the new medicine—clinical experimentation, autopsy, and statistics. The hospital came to be the new frame of reference for medical thinking because it was here that the new medicine could be best applied and confirmed, either in surgery, the patient's bed, or in the autopsy room. The new hospital of the 1790s had a strategic role in the development of the new medicine in France.

During the 1790s, the process began by which French medicine was centralized, simplified, and standardized. Many worthless medicinals, because of wartime shortages, were eliminated from the materia medica. Hygiene was emphasized as never before because of experiences derived from the battlefields and encampments of the mass armies of the Republic. Military medicine produced many superior medical and surgical procedures which were popularized and gradually standardized. The state assumed the full burden of providing adequate health care for all of its citizens, although the realization of this aim was yet a long way off. Hospitals became state-supported and state-operated under uniform national regulations and were transformed increasingly into places for cure and even for the prevention of illness. When the medical schools were finally reestablished, they were staffed by men of proven ability whose approach to medicine was concrete and the standardized curriculum reflected the practical experience of the war years.

From 1792 to 1796, virtually all aspects of French medicine were harnessed to the war effort. The story of the military medical service during this period is that of a tremendous contribution and powerful stimulus to the "new medicine" in France. While a few distinguished civilian physicians and surgeons moved ahead with clinical and hospital medicine, the great organizer and diffuser of the new medical knowledge and surgical techniques was the military medical service. Battlefield medicine replaced many old theories with sounder practical experience. The military hospitals became prototypes for improved civilian facilities. Now that talent was supreme, the armies were increasingly served by the ablest men in French medicine and surgery. From a larger viewpoint, the Revolution gave many opportunities to poor boys from the countryside and small towns to study medicine for the first time, and many of them became the men who won later fame as the brilliant physicians and surgeons of the armies of Napoleon and the teachers and great discoverers of the next generation.

Thus the new foundation that had been laid for French medicine and surgery by 1796 was the direct consequence of the trauma of revolution and war. As Ackernecht has pointed out, there is no escaping the irony of a revolutionary movement that set out to eradicate doctors, hospitals, and medical organizations and institutions and ended by creating a new public health policy, more and better doctors, new schools for them, and new and more effective hospitals.[2] When one compares the medical world of 1789 with that of 1796, a great gulf is apparent; the conclusion is inescapable that in those short years, a medical revolution had indeed occurred.

The French Revolution, of course, needs little introduction as the source of many dramatic changes in the world since 1789. The voluminous records of that violent event have led generations of historians to assess and reassess its political, social, and economic ramifications. The medical revolution, however, that occurred in France during these years has been of interest to only a few. Such accepted classic histories of this period as Alphonse Aulard's *Histoire politique de la Révolution*, Georges Lefebvre's

La Révolution française, Albert Mathiez's *La Révolution française*, J. M. Thompson's *French Revolution*, and Crane Brinton's *A Decade of Revolution* contain virtually no mention or recognition of the significant changes in French medicine and their impact upon military, social, and institutional developments. Brinton, my former mentor, did take note of "that common figure, the Jacobin physician" in his study of *The Jacobins*, but quickly passed on to more familiar political events. Other monographs and biographies have skirted the fringes, for example, W. A. Smeaton's *Fourcroy*, McKie's *Lavoisier*, McCloy's trilogy on French inventions, government assistance, and the humanitarian movement,[3] Norman Hampson's *Social History of the French Revolution*, or Joseph Fayet's *La Révolution française et la science*.

The historians of medicine, on the other hand, have tended to concentrate upon the technical and professional achievements of famous French physicians and surgeons, content to leave it to the reader's erudition or imagination to provide an understanding of how they related to the turbulent political and socioeconomic life of their day.[4] Such men as Corvisart, Desault, Sabatier, Pinel or their students Bichat, Laënnec, and Bretonneau are all familiar names in the histories of medicine of this period. Historians of the army medical service have focused, and rightly so, upon the brilliance of Coste, Desgenettes, Larrey, and Percy.[5] Toward an understanding of the professional, institutional, and ideological milieu in which these Frenchmen lived and to which they contributed, other scholars have made really valuable studies, especially Erwin Ackernecht, George Rosen, and Owsei Temkin.[6]

The published documents of the French Revolution have been used by a number of historians to detail how science fared; but these studies, perhaps because the French themselves considered medicine to be an art, have generally ignored the available materials on medicine. Standard documentary sources, if carefully gleaned, yield much information on this subject, especially the *Archives parlementaires* (edited by M. J. Madival and M. E. Laurent, 82 vols., 1862–1919), the *Ancien Moniteur* (32 vols., 1847–50), the *Recueil des actes du Comité de salut public* (edited by Alphonse Aulard, 26 vols., 1889–1923), Bonnal de Ganges's *Les Représentants du peuple en mission près les armées, 1791–1797* (4 vols., 1898), and M. J. Guillaume's editions of the *Procès-verbaux du Comité d'instruction publique de l'Assemblée Législative* (1889) and *Procès-verbaux du Comité d'instruction publique de la Convention nationale* (6 vols., 1891–1904).

Indispensable for reliable information on French medicine and medical men are the 46 volumes of the *Nouvelle biographie* (edited by J. C. F.

Hoefer, 1853–66) and the 100 volumes of the *Dictionnaire encyclopédique des sciences médicales* (1864–89). Good secondary works include those by Augustin Cabanès, Maxime Laignel-Lavastine, and J. Rieux and J. Hassenforder. Biographical studies of value are Paul Triaire's *Larrey et les campaigns de la Révolution et de l'Empire* (1902), André Soubiran's recent *Le Baron Larrey, chirurgien de Napoléon* (1966), and Charles Laurent's *Histoire de la vie et des ouvrages de P. F. Percy* (1827). Published memoirs and studies left by French military medical men who were active in the campaigns of the First Republic are exceptional sources, especially those of Pierre François Briot, Pierre Coze, Charles Louis Dumas, Michel Tennetar, G. G. Lafont-Gouzi, Jacques Cassanyes, Dominique Jean Larrey, and Pierre François Percy.[7]

Most valuable and informative of all are the original documents, handwritten reports, and medical observations of physicians and surgeons, hospital administrators, and medical inspectors, held in Paris in the Archives historique du Service de Santé and in the Musée Val-de-Grâce. The administrative records of the Service historique de l'armée at Vincennes, the resources of the Bibliothèque Nationale, the library of the Faculté de Médecine, and the museum and records at the Invalides shed considerable light upon the whole spectrum of medicine during the revolutionary era.

The need for a synthesis that places medicine in the context of revolution and war during the period from 1789 to 1796 has long existed. This study is an effort to bring together many diverse developments in French life during this period, and to summarize and interpret the interaction between the medical profession and an epoch of far-reaching changes in French society. Actually, the medical revolution that took place in these years constitutes a microcosm of the macrocosm that we call the French Revolution, and each revolution influenced the other. The transformation of institutions under a revolutionary public social philosophy affected the new course of health care for people. New medical approaches and techniques, as well as the new hospital system which emerged from this era, helped to lay the foundation for modern medicine in France. Revolution and war were not only the anvil and hammer that shaped a new France; they helped to forge a new medicine as well.

NOTES

1. Erwin Ackernecht, *Medicine at the Paris Hospital, 1794–1848* (Baltimore, 1967), p.xi.

2. Ibid., p.7.

3. Shelby T. McCloy, *French Inventions of the Eighteenth Century* (Lexington, Ky., 1952); *Government Assistance in Eighteenth-Century France* (Durham, N.C., 1946); and *The Humanitarian Movement in Eighteenth-Century France* (University, Ky., 1957).

4. For example, see Augustin Cabanès, *Les évadés de la médecine* (Paris, 1931); Lester King, *The Medical World of the Eighteenth Century* (Chicago, 1958); and Maxime Laignel-Lavastine, *Histoire générale de la médecine, de la pharmacie, de l'art dentaire, et de la vétérinaire,* 3 vols. (Paris, 1936–49).

5. Good illustrations of this approach are Fielding H. Garrison, *Notes on the History of Military Medicine* (Washington, 1922) and J. Rieux and J. Hassenforder, *Histoire du Service de Santé militaire* (Paris, 1950).

6. Examples of studies by these three prolific writers are Erwin Ackernecht, *Medicine at the Paris Hospital* (Baltimore, 1967); George Rosen, "Hospitals, Medical Care and Social Policy in the French Revolution," *Bulletin of the History of Medicine* 30 (1956): 124–49; and Owsei Temkin, "The Role of Surgery in the Rise of Modern Medical Thought," ibid. 35 (1951): 248–59.

7. Pierre François Briot, *Histoire de l'état et des progrès de la chirurgie militaire en France pendant les guerres de la Révolution* (Besançon, 1817); Pierre Coze, "Mémoire sur la fièvre pretechicale nerveuse qui à régne en Alsace pendant l'hiver de 1791," *Journal de médecine* (Paris, May 1792); Charles Louis Dumas, *Systeme méthodique de nomenclature et de classification des muscles du corps humaine* (Paris, 1797); G. G. Lafont-Gouzi, *Matériaux pour servir à l'histoire de la médecine militaire en France* (Paris, 1809); Pierre Vidal, "Documents inédits: mission de Cassanyes aux armées d'Italie et des Alpes réunies," *La Révolution française* 16: 440–64, 540–66, and "Cassanyes et ses mémoires inédits," ibid. 14: 968–1008; Michel Tennetar, *Traitement de la Dyssenterie qui règne dans le départment de la Moselle (en Septembre 1793)* (Metz, 1793); Pierre François Percy, *Manuel du chirurgien d'armée* (Paris, 1792); and Dominique Jean Larrey, *Recueil de mémoires de chirurgie* (Paris, 1821), *Relation historique et chirurgicale de l'expédition de l'armée d'Orient* (Paris, 1803), *Surgical Essays,* translated by John Rovere (Baltimore, 1823), and *Memoirs of Military Surgery,* translated by R. W. Hall (Baltimore, 1814).

Chapter One

FRENCH MEDICINE
BEFORE THE REVOLUTION

Eighteenth-century medicine was characteristically "library medicine"; that is, it was based upon philosophical theories of illness rather than upon observation and experience. Passing fads and speculative philosophies attributed diseases to "bad humors," weak "vital juices," or to some imbalance of "life forces." John Brown's English school of medical thought stuffed the sick with stimulants while the followers of Holland's Hermann Boerhaave favored giving strong drugs and starving their patients. Von Haller's German-oriented group held to the idea of "irritability" as the basic life function. Théophile Bordeu's Paris-centered entourage preached "harmonious equilibrium" as necessary for health, while Montpellier's Paul Barthez[1] proclaimed a "vitalism" that viewed the human body as a test tube of chemical fermentations, neutralizations, and sublimations. "Iatrochemists" like Barthez bitterly assailed "Iatro-mechanists" for their teaching that man was just an assemblage of pipes, pistons, and pumps, to be dealt with by plumbing methods. There were even those called "Antisystematics" who, as Bordeu scornfully said, "followed a theory of medicine composed of the debris of others," while the fastest growing aggregation of medical men were the "Observers" who, under the influence of Rousseau's ideas, "simply followed Nature."[2]

Profound disillusionment with these quarrelsome philosophies and the inadequacy of traditional medicine helped to produce the phenomenon of Mesmerism in the 1780s. Franz Anton Mesmer, a Viennese physician, capitalized upon the Enlightenment's facination with heat, light, electricity, and magnetism. He came to Paris and captured the popular imagination with his new theory of healing. Sickness resulted, Mesmer said, when some "obstacle" blocked the flow of an invisible "fluid" through the body. This "fluid," which permeated the entire universe, not only explained scientific phenomena; its medical application resulted in restored health. The individual who used Mesmer's tubs, rods, and ropes, massaging his body's "poles," could overcome the obstacle to health by inducing a crisis (often a convulsion) which signaled his cure.[3] Passionate and influential devotees of Mesmerism continued to attract thousands of rabid followers even after a Royal Commission headed by Benjamin Franklin pronounced it a fraud.[4] Boiling over, the Mesmerists published a flood of works defending their cures, and the swelling public interest after 1784 was evidence of "mesmerism's power to entertain, if not cure."[5]

Provincial medicine in France lacked philosophic systems but embraced an extraordinary variety of medieval conceptions and practices. Many otherwise intelligent people thought that the Devil was the author of most afflictions, although they often attributed the plague and cholera to the anger of God. An incredible number of traditional remedies were available locally for minor ailments. Healing by the intercession of the saints was believed and widely claimed. But many of the suffering and desperately sick sought to be cured by magic or by some "great physician," and the countryside was filled with itinerants who peddled exotic elixirs, secret cure-alls, magic remedies, and charm potions.[6]

The elementary principles of sanitation were simply a mystery to most eighteenth-century Frenchmen. Diseases bred freely in polluted streams and in refuse-clogged roads and narrow, puddled streets. Diphtheria, measles, smallpox, and scarlet fever were killers known in every town, but the diagnosis and treatment often failed to correspond to the disease. In rural France especially, epizootics caused more illness than anything else. Every winter and spring, epidemic pneumonias and *la grippe* appeared. Typhoid fever, dysentery, and malaria repeatedly ravaged France during the eighteenth century. People still saw in any epidemic illness the possibility of a return of the bubonic plague, for which the best prescription was simply to "flee quickly, go far, and come back slowly."[7]

Lice and the itch were endemic, affecting practically everyone. The cheapest and most popular cure for the itch (of the thousands of local remedies available) was "Mother's Ointment," a concoction of suet, mutton fat, butter, lard, and lead oxide. A quack remedy of some vogue among the itching was the quicksilver belt, a strip of linen smeared with mercury and white of egg and worn around the waist. To ward off infection of every sort, almost everyone carried some form of personal disinfectant. The most famous, "Four Thieves Vinegar," was highly recommended by physicians.[8]

Venereal disease was prevalent, but no distinction had been made between syphilis and gonorrhea. The infected person's desire for secrecy and his hope for an easy cure supported thousands of amateurs who were engaged in the chemistry of antivenereal potions. "Lisbon Diet Drink,"

"Solar Balm," and "Astral Water" competed with countless other complicated "remedies" in a very lucrative market. A long-standing quarrel as to which was the best treatment, mercury or guaiacum, still raged between their partisans, but Jean Keyser's mercury preparations proved to be the most effective and remained the antivenereal pills used in all French military hospitals.[9]

In eighteenth-century France, an *hôpital* was almost any charitable agency recognized by the state as existing for the benefit of the needy, whether sick, dependent, or disabled. Religious orders operated many of them, especially the provincial and small town institutions known as places of "care" rather than of "cure." City hospitals usually were municipally owned and controlled, and accounted for the greater part of medical charity work in France. The chief hospital in each town was commonly called the Hôtel-Dieu; others were often labeled the Charité or named for a saint. Hospitals were usually deficit operations. Their incomes were derived from a tremendous variety of sources. Only 5 to 10 percent of all hospital revenues came from the Church directly. Principal incomes were from monetary or landed endowment and from a tax, the *octroi*, on various commodities. Alms, fines, feudal dues and fees, sales, and government supplements made up the remainder. Hospitals usually had charity workshops in which idle and needy women could sew, make cloth and lace, and fashion bandages. The sale of mortuary cloth, a hospital monopoly, augmented income. Hospital service was rendered free by many physicians and surgeons, even though such service was often regarded as a sentence of death because of the terrible hospital conditions.[10]

The hospital pharmacy was usually a reflection of the local apothecary shop. During the eighteenth century, rather than simplifying the available medicinals, physicians and surgeons added such controversial new ones as arsenic in solution (aqua Toffana), ipecacuanha, acetate of lead, nitrate of silver, quassia, clematis, senega, castor oil, digitalis, and kino. G. G. Lafont-Gouzi's secret antidysentery potion called for only rhubarb, canella, syrup, and laudanum, but the dentist Pierre Fauchard's popular tooth remedy contained shellac, catechu, rose honey, a Sumatran resin called dragon's blood, cinnamon, pyrethrum, cloves, red sandalwood, bones of black fish, calcined eggshells, and calcined salt.[11] More outlandish prescriptions were not unknown, but rarely did one gain wide acceptance. The apothecary shop usually stocked only time-tested remedies. Amulets, millipedes, wood lice, acorns, mummy, urine, and various kinds of dung were thought to be efficacious and, with a tremendous number of other popular ingredients, could be found in the average apothecary's shop. The physician's prescriptions continued to be prepared by methods centuries old so that the pharmacy in eighteenth-century France "still resembled a witches' kitchen."[12]

Standard practice required the physician to reveal his secret potion's ingredients only to the apothecary (by the usual symbols meaningless to laymen). It was also common for extravagant claims to be made for the efficacy of one's remedy. "Hemithochorton," presented to the Royal Society of Medicine in 1778, was said by its sponsor to be good for "verminous illnesses, putrid fevers, irregular fevers, convulsions, colics, pleurisy, coughs, whooping cough, abdominal inflammation, epilepsy, dysentery, acute colic in new-born infants."[13]

The bladder stone was by far the greatest affliction of ordinary Frenchmen who needed surgery. All accounts of eighteenth-century French medicine refer to the excruciating pain of the stone and to the swarms of itinerant lithotomists who swept through the countryside leaving a trail of dead and dying in their wake. There were also barbers, barber-surgeons, surgeon-barbers, and surgeon-dentists who operated in the villages and towns. Fame and fortune awaited the knife-wielder who performed a successful lithotomy. It was often assumed that anyone could do surgery and the potential rewards induced many to try. The grisly record compiled by amateur lithotomists did not deter the people from flocking to them, preferring mutilation and even death to the unendurable pain. Ignorant operatives, by slashing through the abdomen and the peritoneum, let men trade their bladder stones for deadly peritonitis. A more cautious few continued to approach the bladder from below, but this required skill and patience. Jean Baseilhac (commonly called Frère Côme) developed the idea for the "hidden stone operation." His incision through the rectum met with considerable success, and Baseilhac quickly moved to Paris to capitalize upon his skill.[14]

Although the Paris surgeons had adopted the scalpel and discarded the razor as "an instrument dishonorable to their science," those of the countryside still used it for tradition's sake and "because their work was less specialized, they found it profitable."[15] There was scarcely any ailment for which "bleeding" was not prescribed, and the surgeons and barbers monopolized this art. Some of them also specialized as rupture surgeons, for rupture was very common among the peasants. Others entered the criminal but very lucrative practice of making *castrati* for the opera or of castrating boys who wished to avoid military service.[16]

The town surgeon was still an artisan who had been apprenticed to his father or to an uncle, while the town physician had had some humanistic education and some introduction to special medicine and medico-technical aspects of knowledge. The surgeon was easily recognizable in his serge vest, fitted waistcoat, and skintight knee breeches, walking to his patient's home "with his silver-trimmed hat on his head, from time to time taking from his pocket his snuffbox of Santa Lucia wood."[17] Despite his pretensions, the surgeon was outshone by the physician. No longer did the physician ride a mule like his seventeenth-century predecessor; he was carried in a sedan chair or driven in a carriage. He had adopted the dress of the wealthy bourgeoisie: a high-ruff collar, a pleated vest, a jacket with gold-lace-trimmed pockets and cuffs, a black fur-trimmed robe of brocade or silk, and a curled, white-powdered wig, queued, ornamented, and separated into layers. His other trademarks were the muff, the pipe, and a gold-headed cane.[18]

Most physicians had gone to the cities in the eighteenth century and were rarely seen by the masses except when some epidemic forced the local authorities to appeal for outside medical help. In such times, the king sent out his top physicians with free medical supplies for epidemic or disaster relief. Local medical practitioners were usually upset. Most of the imported physicians refused any pay and insisted that everyone should labor free, though some of them profiteered and drained money from local clients. Most infuriating of all was their unbearable haughtiness and contempt for the local practitioner. However, his wounded pride was usually salved by the reluctance of the peasants to receive the government physicians and, more exasperatingly, their unwillingness to follow the prescribed remedies.[19]

In the cities, physicians, surgeons, and apothecaries were formed into medieval associations carrying various names (*communauté, collège, compagnie*), regulated themselves, and had representation through their elected guild delegates. In the social scale, physicians ranked above surgeons and surgeons above apothecaries, but all three belonged generally to the Third Estate and, with a few exceptions, were in the three lowest pension groups—one-half of them in the very lowest.[20]

The social and professional prestige of the physician in eighteenth-century France stemmed from varied sources. First of all, he was usually university trained, something the surgeon or apothecary could rarely boast. Also, medical practice was considered by laymen as the pursuit of a conscientious vocation, not a business or a craft. Nor were physicians too plentiful for their own independence and prestige. For example, in a population of 32,000 at Rennes there were but five physicians, "for the needs of the rich."[21] About this same ratio was evident as late as 1792 in Paris, which had 139 physicians and 171 surgeons for its 610,000 inhabitants.[22]

The physician was the family doctor; when his patient was ill, other healers came only as advisors or technicians. Sebastien Mercier, who hated physicians, said that "no one dares contradict the orders of the presiding physician and the patient dies in the midst of ten doctors, who see very well what ought to be done to save him but who, by *esprit de corps*, let the first-called . . . effect his methodical assassination."[23] There was never any doubt as to who was in charge: the family physician dominated the surgeon-barber and the apothecary too. A medical trinity had already been established. The physician diagnosed and prescribed. The surgeon routinely bled the patient. The apothecary filled the prescriptions, and since "purging was as popular as eating and drinking," he also administered the enema.[24] The solidarity of these three was summarized in Cyrano de Bergerac's quip: "As soon as they enter the room, one sticks out his tongue to the doctor, turns his backside to the apothecary and extends his arm to the barber."[25]

It was very difficult for a physician to build a practice. People rarely changed physicians and medical practice was commonly attained by a kind of inheritance from a relative, family friend, or by the recommendation of an older, respected physician. Because the institution of the family priest was dying as the century wore on, the physician came to occupy a secure place in the family as a confidant and friend. Those who were attached to families of the nobility and the well-to-do middle class enjoyed regular stipends and did not have to ask pay for their professional services. The towns also often engaged physicians for an annual salary to give free medical service to the poor. Physicians not so fortunately provided for, however, followed an old French proverb (*il refuse d'une main qui le voudrait tenir de l'autre*) by hypocritically waving away a proferred fee with one hand while holding the other out behind him to take it. The popular Paris physician Antoine Portal made 43,000 francs in 1788, but "the average practitioner could, at best, charge one-fourth of what the princes of the profession demanded."[26]

In Paris, the mecca of French medicine, prestige was often measured by dress and gadgets. The popular physicians carried in their pockets silver bleeding cups (the new artificial leeches).[27] The very rich specialist on gas and vapors, Pierre Pomme, was "a dandy doctor with a very fine figure, good talker, dressed very elegantly and correctly in order to seduce the ladies."[28] Paul Barthez used a gold-decorated tourniquet when bleeding the ladies. Some individuals like Antoine Lorry, "all covered with ribbons, silks and perfumes," were known for their outlandish costumes. Théophile de Bordeu visited his patients in the mornings in a reddish-gray robe of cloth-of-gold; in the evenings he was "muskratted and silvered."[29] Nicolas Corvisart was one of the few who kept his natural hair, but it cost him a position in the hospital founded by Madame Necker, who told him that "the place would be given only to a doctor who wore a wig."[30] Théodore Tronchin was one of the rare ones to maintain austere dress, "owing to the gravity of his position" as physician to the Duc d'Orléans.[31]

Small provincial universities continued to supply the medical profession with physicians trained purely in theoretical medicine, but few of them ever made it beyond the small towns and cities as practitioners. These graduates evidenced much dissatisfaction with their training as the Revolution drew near. Students during the 1780s became increasingly vocal and bitter over the incongruity of a professor who lectured on chemical theory but scorned the drudgery of doing an experiment or soiling his hands with chemicals. A young medical student, Jacques Cassanyes, wrote home in disgust that a local nobleman was acting as the anatomy demonstrator at the University of Perpignan. The demonstrator, François Xavier de Llucia, was a very rich man who had no desire to practice medicine or surgery but simply wished to know some anatomy and satisfy his curiosity about the human body.[32] More outrageous to all was the fact that a professor's "demonstrator," in performing what the professor had just theorized, often proved just the opposite. So poor was medical instruction that few saw anything amiss in the way in which some men entered the profession. The colorful Anthelme Brillat-Savarin simply announced himself as "an amateur physician," and after his famous treatise on the digestive system had made him a foremost authority by 1776, he calmly gave himself a master's degree and the title of Professor.[33] On June 30, 1775, the University of Saint-André d'Ecosse (Eure) even awarded Jean Paul Marat the degree of Doctor of Medicine, "a sort of honorary title, delivered on the recommendation of two known physicians," for which Marat did not have to pass any examination.[34]

At the old established universities like Montpellier and Paris, the traditional theological and philosophical approach to medical learning had turned them into what some called "bastions of learned ignorance."[35] Champions of Hippocrates and Galen, entrenched in the faculties, quarreled endlessly over the effectiveness of chinchona, the use of antimony, and the circulation of the blood. Jean Antoine Chaptal recorded that he became so devoted to disputation that he always took the opposite side of any thesis brought up at Montpellier. He even ruined a friend's doctoral examination through his egotistical devotion to argument.[36] Faculty doctors like Chaptal seemed to many Frenchmen to epitomize the stagnation of medical knowledge. Because the doctors would not jeopardize their teaching positions by attempting to practice, clinical medicine was largely unknown to them.

The most formidable opponent of change and medical advance was the Faculty of Medicine of the University of Paris. For six hundred years it had enjoyed wide privileges and powerful monopolies. The doctors of the College of Surgery of Saint Côme had acquired independence from it only after a bitter struggle. For a long time, these two faculties alone could authorize one to practice medicine or surgery in Paris. Until early in the French Revolution, the Faculty of Medicine had the exclusive right to grant the degree of *docteur régent*, a requirement for a teaching position in the Paris medical schools.[37]

The founding of the Royal Academy of Surgery on December 8, 1731, had begun the reduction of the monopolistic privileges of the Saint Côme faculty. Surgeons were emancipated from their control twelve years later. Louis XV's famous Ordinance of April 23, 1743, separated surgeons from the Company of Barbers, awarded them the same privileges as the doctors of Saint Côme, gave them rights to the Master of Arts degree, and raised surgery to the rank of a liberal profession.[38]

The Paris Faculty of Medicine was not shaken until the Royal Society of Medicine was founded on August 13, 1776. Then the Paris Faculty charged infringement upon its rights, peititioned the crown bitterly, and finally threatened with expulsion any Paris Faculty member who joined the new Royal Society. It could win but two concessions from the crown: two-thirds of the Royal Society's associate membership was reserved for Paris Faculty members, and the Royal Society agreed to meet with the Paris Faculty semiannually to inform them of current discoveries, new research, and the general progress of medicine. However, the Paris Faculty still controlled teaching in the medical schools. It refused, as late as 1780, to grant the degree of *docteur régent* to Antoine Fourcroy, even though he raised the necessary fee of 6,000 livres, on the grounds that he had kept the books of the rival Academy of Sciences during his student days.[39] In that same year, Claude Berthollet, the protégé of Tronchin, entered the Academy of Sciences, but he was still required to prepare another medical thesis to satisfy the Paris Faculty.[40]

It is no wonder that most eighteenth-century Frenchmen seemed convinced of the truth of the famous ceremony in Molière's *Le Malade imaginaire*. In that comedy the doctoral candidate's solution to every medical question was always *"Clysterium donare, postea seignare, ensuitta purgare"* ("Give a clyster, then bleed, then purge"); and the highly satisfied faculty chanted in chorus at each reply *" Bene, bene, bene, bene respondare, dignus, dignus est entrare in nostro docto corpore"*

("Excellently, excellently, excellently answered; worthy, worthy is he to enter into our learned company").[41] Most Parisians knew that when a license to practice in Paris was conferred, even on the eve of the Revolution this old formula was still intoned: *"Ego, cancellarius, auctoritate apostolica, qua druor in hac parte, do vobis licentiam legendi, interpretandi, et faciendi medicinam hic et ubique terrarum. In nomine Patris, et Fili, et Spiritu Sancti"* ("I, the Chancellor, by the power invested by the apostolic authority which I exercise in these parts, confer on you the faculty to teach, to interpret, and to practice medicine, here and in all countries. In the name of the Father, the Son, and the Holy Spirit").[42] The faculty doctors still seemed to be able to shrug off all criticism and satire in the cynical fashion of the seventeenth century's Jean de la Bruyère: "As long as men must die and as long as they love to live, physicians will be a special breed and well paid."[43]

The climate of the eighteenth century was different from that of Molière's time; there was no "genial spirit" to soften the sting of contemporary criticism of monopolistic and faulty medical practices.[44] Denis Diderot, writing in the *Encyclopédie*, noted that one's health returned more easily "if the faculty is not involved in it."[45] In his popular *Emile*, Jean Jacques Rousseau's boast was emphatic: "I swear that never having called a physician for myself, I will never call one for Emile." Voltaire's observation held real venom: "One who is destined to be struck by apoplexy is also destined to find a wise physician, who bleeds him, purges him, and permits him to live until the fatal moment." The impatience of the Enlightenment was manifest in Condorcet's charge that medicine was committed to "false theories, to its pedantic jargon, to its murderous routine, to its servile submission to the authority of men, to doctrines of faculties; it understands neither how to think nor to experiment."[46]

NOTES

1. Barthez dossier, carton 204 B/1, Musée Val-de-Grâce, Paris (hereinafter cited as Val-de-Grâce). In the Val-de-Grâce museum in Paris, the dossiers of documents on individual military physicians and surgeons are filed in alphabetical order in numbered cartons.

2. Constant Hillemand, "Histoire de la médecine," *Le progrès médicale* 47, no.40 (1932): 1662; Richard R. Mathison, *The Eternal Search: The Story of Man and His Drugs* (New York, 1958), p.283; Douglas McKie, *Antoine Lavoisier: Scientist, Economist, Social Reformer* (New York 1952), pp.167ff.; W. A. Smeaton, *Fourcroy, Chemist and Revolutionary, 1755–1809* (Cambridge, 1962), pp.10ff.

3. Robert Darnton, *Mesmerism and the End of the Enlightenment in France* (Cambridge, Mass., 1968), pp.4–8.

4. Benjamin Franklin, *Report of Benjamin Franklin and Other Commissioners Charged by the King of France with the Examination of the Animal Magnetism* (London, 1785), passim.

5. Darnton, *Mesmerism*, pp.38–41, 52.

6. Hillemand, "Histoire de la médecine," *Progrès médicale* 47: 1658.

7. The bubonic plague continued to ravage eastern Europe, although the last major outbreak in France occurred in 1720. Johann H. Baas, *Outlines of the History of Medicine and the Medical Profession* (New York, 1889), pp.628–29; Mathison, *Eternal Search*, p.202.

8. The itch was a term that often covered cankerrash, impetigo, eczema, or any skin irritation caused by arachnids. Baas, *Outlines* pp.653–54; McCloy, *Government Assistance*, p.145.

9. Guaiacum, often called the "Remedy of the Caribs," was popular in the sixteenth century, but it was ineffective for syphilis. It was derived from the guyac tree found principally in Jamaica. *Dictionnaire de médecine* 14: 30; Abraham Wolf, *A History of Science, Technology, and Philosophy in the Eighteenth Century* (London, 1952), p.497; Laignel-Lavastine, *Histoire générale* 2: 536–40.

10. In 1787, there were more than one hundred young surgeons who, in order to learn, gave free service at the Hôtel-Dieu in Paris. By tradition, the Hôtel-Dieu of Lyon financed its indigent care by requiring each of the administrators to advance 100,000 livres and the total was invested to produce an annual income. Each new administrator reimbursed his predecessor, thus maintaining this endowment at a steady level. M. J. Madival and M. E. Laurent, eds., *Archives parlementaires de 1787 à 1860. Recueil complet des débats législatifs et politiques des chambres françaises*, 82 vols. (Paris, 1862–1919), 42: 582 (hereinafter cited as *Arch. parl.*); Garrison, *Notes*, p.155; McCloy, *Government Assistance*, pp.181, 187, 236.

11. Carton 107, Archives historiques de Service de Santé militaire, Paris (hereinafter cited as Arch. Service de Santé). In the Archives historiques du Service de Santé militaire in Paris, the documents are filed in numbered cartons according to subject and have been indexed by Jean Bonnerot, *La bibliothèque centrale et les archives du Service de Santé* (Paris, 1918). Gabriel Gregoire Lafont-Gouzi (1777—1850) of Saverdun (Arriège). See Lafont-Gouzi, *Matériaux*, p.131, and B. W. Weinberger, *Pierre Fauchard* (Minneapolis, 1941), p.66.

12. Baas, *Outlines*, p.725.

13. M. J. Guillaume, ed., *Procès-verbaux du Comité d'instruction publique de la Convention nationale*, 6 vols. (Paris, 1891—1904), 2: 140—41 (hereinafter cited as *Convention*).

14. Jurgen Thorwald, *The Century of the Surgeon* (New York, 1957), pp.31—35; McCloy, *French Inventions*, p.155.

15. M. B. Paumes, "La parenté médicale du maréchal Bessières," *Chronique médicale* 20: 193—96 (hereinafter cited as *Chron. méd.*).

16. An army recruiting officer, J. L. Fourcroy, in 1775 reported one surgeon who castrated seventeen boys in one day in a small town near Clermont. Fourcroy swore that in one morning he "counted 46 castrates out of 160 youths who reported" to his recruiting table. McCloy, *Humanitarian Movement*, p.212.

17. Augustin Cabanès, *Le costume du médecin en France de Molière à nos jours* (Paris, n.d.), p.33.

18. Augustin Cabanès, *La médecine en caricature* (Paris, n.d.), p.14.

19. Laignel-Lavastine, *Histoire générale* 3: 726; McCloy, *Government Assistance*, pp.144, 163.

20. *Arch. parl.* 13: 322; Laignel-Lavastine, *Histoire générale* 3: 553—54, 726; McCloy, *Government Assistance*, p.273. The rank of physicians on the economic scale was reflected by the Paris "poor tax" (an *octroi* on wine) which assessed artisans at 13 sous, physicians at 16 sous, and lawyers at 52 sous.

21. Baas, *Outlines*, p.731; Garrison, *Notes*, p.152; J. M. Thompson, *The French Revolution* (New York, 1945), p.72.

22. Auguste Corlieu, *Le centenaire de la Faculté de Médecine de Paris* (Paris, 1896), pp.3—4.

23. Sebastien Mercier (1740—1814), French journalist and revolutionary, quoted in Augustin Cabanès, *Médecins amateurs* (Paris, 1932), p.311.

24. Mathison, *Eternal Search*, p.220.

25. Sarinien de Cyrano de Bergerac (1619—c.1655) of Paris, famous French man of letters, quoted in Cabanès, *Caricature*, p.20.

26. Ackernecht, *Paris Hospital*, p.115; Paul Delaunay, *D'une révolution à l'autre, 1789—1848* (Paris, 1949), p.34.

27. Charles J. S. Thompson, *The History and Evolution of Surgical Instruments* (New York, 1942), pp.82—83. Ladies often objected to being

bled by having live leeches attached to the skin and preferred the bleeding cups which were fitted with numerous needles for puncturing the skin.

28. Pierre Pomme (1735–1812) of Arles. Cabanès, *Costume*, p.32.

29. Paul Joseph Barthez (1734–1806) of Montpellier taught the importance of glandular functions and pioneered the theory of internal secretions. Barthez dossier, carton 204 B/1, Val-de-Graĉe. Antoine Lorry (1725–83) of Paris concluded that the medulla was the seat of vital functions and anticipated Flourens in localizing the medulla as the center of respiration, J. C. F. Hoefer, ed., *Nouvelle biographie*, 46 vols. (Paris, 1853–66), 31: 688.

30. Jean Nicolas Corvisart des Marets (1755–1821) of Dricourt (Ardennes) studied in Paris under Desault, Pelletan, and Hallé, and used percussion (Auenbrugger's discovery of the validity of tapping the chest with the fingers) in teaching students at the Charité. He was physician to Barras during the Revolution and later First Physician to Napoleon I and a Baron of the Empire. Corvisart dossier, carton 205/1, Val-de-Graĉe.

31. Théodore Tronchin (1709–81), a Swiss physician, First Physician to the Duc d'Orléans and to Louis XVI. Noted for his fresh air and exercise fads which he popularized in Paris. *Nouvelle biographie* 45: 665; Cabanès, *Costume*, p.32.

32. Vidal, "Cassanyes," *Révolution française* 14: 985.

33. Jean Anthelme Brillat-Savarin (1755-1826) of Belley (Ain), member of the Estates-General and National Assembly. During the Reign of Terror he emigrated to New York. See Maxime Brienne, "Brillat-Savarin," *Chron. méd.* 28: 323; Maurice Genty, "Brillat-Savarin," *Progrès médicale* 34: 386; and Armand de Lagnieu, "La médecin dans Brillat-Savarin," ibid., 36: 433–34.

34. Joseph Fayet, *La Révolution française et la science, 1789–1795* (Paris, 1960), p.28n.

35. Leo Gershoy, *From Despotism to Revolution, 1763–1789* (New York, 1963), p.275.

36. George Rosen and Beate Caspari-Rosen, *400 Years of a Doctor's Life* (New York, 1947), p.61. Jean Antoine Chaptal (1756–1832) of Nogaret (Lozére), *Nouvelle biographie* 9: 706–9.

37. M. Boutry, "La médecine et les institutions charitables au temps de Louis XVI," *Chron. méd.* 11: 742; Jean des Cilleuls, "Les médecins aux armées d'ancien régime," *Revue historique de l'armées* 6: 10; McKie, *Lavoisier*, pp.72–73.

38. In England at about this time (1745) a group of surgeons seceded from the Company of Barber-Surgeons and formed the Corporation of Surgeons. See John Kobler, *The Reluctant Surgeon: The Life of John Hunter* (London, 1960), p.36, and Laignel-Lavastine, *Histoire générale* 2: 437, 441; 3: 724.

39. Boutry, "La médecine," *Chron. méd.* 11: 742; Smeaton, *Fourcroy*, pp.2–5.

40. "C", "Quelques évadés," *Chron. méd.* 30: 99. Claude Louis Berthollet (1748–1822) of Savoy, distinguished chemist, aided the Committee of Public Safety in mobilizing for war. Later, he was a Count of the Empire. *Dictionnaire encyclopédique des sciences médicales*, 100 vols. (Paris, 1864–89), 1st ser., 9: 181.

41. Turgeon and Gilligan, eds., *The Principal Comedies of Molière* (New York, 1947), p.1031.

42. Milton I. Roemer, ed., *Henry E. Sigerist on the Sociology of Medicine* (New York, 1960), p.313.

43. Jean de la Bruyère (1639–96), French moralist and author, quoted in René Cruchet, *Médecine et littérature* (University, La., 1939), p.171.

44. Cruchet insists upon the "genial spirit" of all of the caricatures and barbs aimed at physicians in Molière's time and says that, when the curtain fell and the farce was played, the audience understood this spirit. Ibid., p.190.

45. Quoted in Cabanès, *Médecins amateurs*, p.182.

46. Rousseau, Voltaire, and Condorcet are quoted in Cruchet, *Médecine et littérature* pp.223, 230, 232.

Chapter Two

REFORM AND CHANGE:
MILITARY MEDICINE AND THE HOSPITALS

The popularity of science in late eighteenth-century France drew men and women alike into medical discussions and amateur practice. Everywhere the salons were crowded, journals gave novel ideas wide publicity, wealthy individuals awarded prizes for new discoveries and "a public elegant and choice" attended the informal lectures of great practicing surgeons and physicians. Even the ladies visited the laboratories, helping with "experiments" and frequently contributing to the popular journals of science and medicine.[1]

The energy and enthusiasm of this prerevolutionary movement welled up from sources much deeper than the many fashionable salons. Founded upon a growing conviction that life should mean happiness for man and constructed of some reinforcing and interlocking ideas about the social utility of reason, enlightenment, and scientific and technological progress, much serious thought about reform focused upon the urgent need to deal effectively with problems of health care and poverty. When in 1788 each electoral assembly in France was authorized to draw up an address of complaints to the crown (*cahier des doléances*) in preparation for the meeting of the Estates-General, these *cahiers* reflected how well various reform programs had been popularized and how deeply many Frenchmen wanted a better life. They also revealed the overwhelming conviction that poverty and sickness lay at the roots of other social problems. General agreement was evident upon the proposition that, for happiness, health was essential.[2] Therefore the grinding poverty of a great part of the French people was directly linked to their diseases and afflictions, the health-destroying trades at which many men were forced to work, ill health from malnutrition, the high infant mortality rate, the inadequacy of medical aid, and the ineffectiveness of the eighteenth-century medical profession.

For a long time it had been a basic principle in France that each community should provide care for its own poor, sick, and afflicted. The Church, charitable organizations, and private individuals contributed to this care, while the crown stepped in substantially only when epidemics or other disasters proved to be too much for the local authorities to handle. The failure of existing private charities and local agencies to deal adequately with the growing problems of poverty and health care became obvious as the eighteenth century matured. One key factor in this failure was that not only was there a shortage of medical personnel to deal with epidemics but a critical lack of qualified physicians, surgeons, and midwives for the ordinary medical needs of the population. Another was the obvious lack of confidence in French medicine as it was being taught and practiced. Even the few Frenchmen who might have been willing to support a costly program of improved health care for the masses felt frustrated by the monopolistic faculties, the poor quality of medical and surgical training, the inadequacy of hospital facilities, and the demonstrated failure of local responsibility. Thus one of the powerful driving forces for change drew strength not only from the poor masses demanding better health care but also from educated, sensitive people who had become convinced that such medical attention was an obligation of society, to be carried out by the national government.[3]

The crown had shown itself capable of movement during the eighteenth century in one significant agency of health care, the military medical service. To many, medical men and laymen alike, the military medical service was a vivid illustration of what a comprehensive, centralized program of medical care might do. The Corps de Santé militaire had been created by Louis XIV. His edict of January 17, 1708, established military hospitals in 51 French cities, specified that sick and wounded soldiers be attended by qualified physicians and surgeons, and set up a hierarchy of medical personnel under the supervision of his First Physician, First Surgeon, and Minister of War.[4] The purchase of positions by physicians and surgeons was stopped in 1716 and a training program established for young surgeons in the military hospitals.[5] On December 20, 1718, the crown issued a document containing the first uniform code of military hospital regulations. It clearly outlined the relation between hospital administrators and the medical personnel, the duties of medical personnel, the treatment of patients, methods of controlling contagious diseases, and elementary rules of hygiene.[6] The administration of military medicine thereafter became a definite function of the government.

Regular inspections and uniform regulations helped to make peacetime military medicine superior to ordinary civilian medicine. The Ordinance of

January 1, 1747, introduced "war commissioners" who made regular inspections of the hospitals, especially to insure that the crown was not being charged for the care of nonexistent patients. This same decree gave official status to apothecaries and fixed their place in the medical service. It also contained uniform regulations for all military hospitals.[7]

The personal hygiene of the soldier was the subject of intensive study in the mid eighteenth century, and several classic works appeared. *Observations on the Diseases of the Army* by John Pringle had a tremendous impact upon Europe, inspiring that same year (1752) a French order requiring that all hospitals whitewash walls to control vermin, have the whole hospital area swept daily, see that the kitchens, pantries, and bakeries were kept clean, and clean all wards twice daily—before wound-dressing time and after the evening meal. Gerard van Swieten's *Diseases Incident to Armies* was so popular that it ran through several European printings; even an American edition appeared in 1776. Too numerous to mention were the studies on venereal disease control. The army had already settled upon a way to handle this acute problem by tolerating "regulated" camp followers, who constituted a sort of "sexual canteen." Besides, most military hospitals in France had special isolation wards for treating infected soldiers with Keyser's mercury remedy, which was the best available anywhere.[8]

The celebrated *Oeconomical and Medical Observations* by Richard Brocklesby (1764) introduced barracks into French military life and fostered improvement of latrines and camps. Food rations were standardized and more serviceable uniforms began to replace theatrical and unsanitary dress. Pringle had a French counterpart, Jean Colombier, who brought out his five-volume *Code de médecine militaire* in 1772, wherein "all that pertained to the well or the sick soldier, in the field, or in the garrison, and to hospitals, army diseases, duties of the military physician, etc." were exhaustively treated.[9]

Ambroise Paré (1552) had attacked vigorously the prevailing notion that gunshot wounds were poisoned, but it still lingered into the eighteenth century; so did "sympathetic powder" and weapon salve designed to neutralize the poison.[10] Fingers were still often used as probes, and even simple wounds were coated with assorted complicated balms, greasy ointments, and perfumed washes used for cleaning wounds. A styptic in standard use was lycoperdon powder, but the treatment of a serious hemorrhage was badly understood. The cautery iron was still used on wounds, even beneficially at times. Wound excision was a precept derived from the notion that healing was promoted by changing the shape of the wound and the belief that a wound that bled little always produced complications. These ideas encouraged surgeons to make several incisions to help a wound bleed and to leave it bleeding a bit or to ring it with leeches. Bleeding and purging of the wound were so routine and so murderous that the Prince de Ligne once cried that he could save his army "if they would permit me to hang the first doctor whom I saw . . . bleed with his right [hand] and purge with his left."[11]

Many surgeons deliberately left soldiers who bled very little to the last, preferring to dress those wounds bleeding freely first because, they reasoned, the former needed time to bleed some more. If this was not voluntarily done, the surgeon usually opened the wound with his knife. As no distinction was made in types of wounds, this concept of treatment often caused grave or irreparable injury to the victim. Gunshot wounds normally were stuffed with lint soaked in "Four Thieves Vinegar," wine, "harquebusade water" or brandy, although stronger antiseptics (tincture of myrrh, camphor, balsam of Peru, or hot turpentine) were used if infection threatened. The ignorance displayed in dealing with wounds made by firearms fortunately had not persisted with other types. By the 1780s, it was deemed sufficient to clean a simple sabre, sword, or bayonet wound, draw the edges together with a suture, and give the wound plenty of air.[12]

Military medicine afforded many opportunities for improvisation and bold inventiveness, especially in wartime. The armed services therefore reaped a harvest of advances not immediately available in civilian practice. Fancy "bow saws," popular in clinical surgery, were replaced in military practice by the "tenon saw" (similar to the carpenter's saw) because of its rugged, simple construction and its proven superiority.[13] The distinguished military surgeon Jean Petit invented an artery forceps and a screw tourniquet, although the *garotte* was still commonly used.[14] Jean Perret's *pince à pansement* (dressing forceps) became a standard military item, as did an artery-compression forceps constructed by Pierre Desault in 1787. Desault also invented a bandage that bears his name, designed to hold an arm correctly in case of a broken collarbone.[15] Various contraptions for setting broken bones were invented, such as the famous "tin boot" of Hugues Ravaton. Antoine Louis developed several types of surgical scissors and a standard amputation knife. Pierre Percy at the outset of the Revolution perfected his *tribulcon*, a bullet extractor hopefully offered as a substitute for fingers.[16]

An ambulance service was created in 1772 to connect the armies with permanent military hospitals. It was also responsible for evacuating wounded to more remote interior hospitals as front-line facilities became overtaxed. Before the Revolution, ambulances were heavy four-wheeled wagons drawn by up to 46 horses. One of these mobile hospitals was assigned to each army of 20,000 men and, based upon experience, it was equipped to handle 2,000 men (one-tenth of the effectives). Its personnel included a surgeon-major, 12 surgeon aides-major, 30 student surgeons, and 30 attendants. In addition to a number of physicians there was a war commissioner, a director, an assistant director, a cook, a baker, three priests, and assorted helpers—a total of 134 men.[17] The French military surgeon, Jacques Bagieu, described the system still in use on the eve of the Revolution, explaining that: "During wartime there is an ambulance hospital more or less within reach of the place where an engagement occurs, where the surgeon-major and other surgeons hold themselves in readiness. This is the first depot where wounded are collected, from whence they are carried to cities farther removed as these become crowded. It is rare that surgical operations are performed in the field proper, that is, at the place where wounds are inflicted, and still more rare[ly] are amputations performed."[18]

Notable efforts had been made to improve the quality of military medicine through the creation of an instructional program within the military system. Although not well enforced, the Ordinance of January 1, 1747, had required that the physician-in-chief of each hospital give a course in medicine and that surgeons-major demonstrate operations and teach anatomy every year during the winter. Special schools, called ampitheaters, were created in 1775 at the regional hospitals at Lille, Metz, and Strasbourg, and shortly thereafter at Brest and Toulon.[19] The top physicians and surgeons of the army and navy taught at these schools, offering a well-defined and comprehensive curriculum in medicine, surgery, and pharmacy. The period of study was a minimum of three years, a maximum of six. Students selected by army recruiters for their ability ("principal students") had to have previously attended the courses of a university faculty or show three years of study with a master surgeon, and pass an examination. Other students, the *élèves bénévoles*, were the sons of army physicians and surgeons admitted so that they could follow their fathers' calling. Some students came from regimental medical service, if they were sponsored by their regiments and recommended by their regimental surgeons-major. At times when the war commissioners and the local intendants agreed, surgeons of the towns and villages were authorized to attend these schools. Here they were trained to be stationed among the troops or in the military hospitals, or placed in reserve and assigned to civilian hospitals.[20]

In the hospitals, a constant, bitter warfare between the war commissioners and the physicians and surgeons raged from 1747 into the early Revolutionary period. Created by the Ordinance of 1747, the nonmedical war commissioners were designed to stop military contractors from defrauding the government. Having "come to do their job, that is, to count the sick and assure themselves that the charges conformed to the actual number of sick men present," the war commissioners quickly won the enmity of medical men, who felt that "little by little, the war commissioners made themselves masters of the service."[21]

The military medical service was also torn by a conflict between physicians and surgeons. The latter found that the physician, just as in civilian life, was dominant and favored in the army. Physicians were not subject to the same discipline that surgeons were. Candidates for "student surgeon" in the army were not examined by the surgeon inspector-general but by the physician inspector-general. Physicians could enter the medical schools without any examination, but surgeons and apothecaries, although products of the same ampitheaters attended by physicians, had to submit proof of studies and to pass examinations. The new hospital code appended to the Ordinance of 1780 placed the physician at the top of each grade, his pay exceeding that of surgeons of the same rank, and seemed to confirm the dominance of physicians over all other medical officers. Therefore, on the eve of the Revolution the whole medical service was looking for an abolition of the hated war commissioners, and surgeons were pressing vigorously to be recognized as equals of the physicians.[22]

The prerevolutionary vitality and brilliance of military medicine was proved by many of its illustrious products. Destined for fame in the wars of the Revolutionary and Napoleonic eras were ampitheater-trained men like P. E. Lafosse, the distinguished military veterinarian; J. A. Lorentz, first physician at the Strasbourg hospital after 1779; and J. F. Coste, chief army physician in 1789. The surgeons included the great Pierre Percy, a regimental surgeon-major at Strasbourg in 1789; Nicolas Saucerotte, an eminent neurologic surgeon and surgeon-major of the French *gendarmerie* in 1789; and others such as Pierre Coze, Charles Louis Dumas, Pierre Gorcy, C. A. Lombard, Jean Thomassin, and Nicolas Heurteloup.[23]

Most distinguished of the great ampitheater-trained teachers were Antoine Louis, permanent secretary of the Academy of Surgery; Raphael Sabatier, anatomist and surgeon-major in 1789 at the Invalides; their more famous student Pierre Desault, professor in the School of Practical Surgery and, after 1785, surgeon-in-chief at the Paris Hôtel-Dieu; Jean Nicolas Corvisart, physician at the Charité in 1788; and Pierre Sue, anatomist in the Paris School of Surgery.[24] As teachers in the medical schools, in the hospitals, and in the free chairs of the private lycées, these men generally stood aloof from the mania for formal "theories" and philosophical "systems" and devoted themselves to clinical medicine and surgery.

The new popular interest in experimental medicine resulted in the creation of hospital-connected schools for more formal training rather than the superficial satisfaction of curiosity. The Estates of Brittany partially supported free surgical schools founded at Rennes in 1748 and at Nantes in 1760. At the Charity Hospital in Grénoble, a religious order began free surgical instruction in 1771.

Other medical schools connected with hospitals sprang up at Brest, at Aix in Provence, at Montpellier, and at Paris. The latter three received some government support and also offered free study opportunities.[25] In 1774, the crown established at Paris a six-bed Hospital of the School of Surgery, endowed it with a professorship in chemistry, an annual income of 7,000 livres, and a laboratory where the faculty and students could keep both men and women patients for special observation and treatment. Struggling against opposition from the doctors of Saint Côme, this beginning of clinical surgery was kept alive and expanded by Pichault de la Martinière, who personally endowed ten more beds in 1782. The following year, as a memorial to him, Louis XVI added another 7,000 livres annual income, six more beds, and a professorship in botany.[26]

Broader opportunities for men in the medical profession began to be realized through the new Academy of Surgery and the Society of Medicine. Both were organized to include provincial members, "free" associates (prominent men in nonmedical fields), and an unlimited number of "correspondents." The latter were practitioners in virtually every town in France and in some foreign countries. They could consult the Academy or the Society, as the case required, on problems encountered in practice, and through these two organizations they could trade advice and information with others in the profession. In turn, the Academy of Surgery and the Society of Medicine gave free instructions and opinions on diseases and operations and set up annual prizes for solutions to medical and surgical problems.[27]

Among those concerned with medical reform during the 1780s there was a curious ambivalence toward hospitals. The health care situation in many hospitals was so disastrous, easy delusions about what could be done privately outside the hospitals were so numerous, and the tendency of politicians to control the government's aid money was so widespread, that some serious reformers like De Chamousset or Dupont de Nemours actually called for the abolition of all hospitals.[28] Typical of the proposed alternative, for instance, was a private *maison de santé* operated during the 1780s near the Sèvre gate in Paris in a spacious courtyard, where the patients were treated at much less cost and were lodged in private or semiprivate rooms. Also notable along this line was the project of the Le Mans philanthropist Joseph Dariot, who cared for 40 sick-poor in a neighboring house while the town surgeon saw them daily without charge (Dariot paid him an annual stipend).[29]

Others, convinced that such private, philanthropic efforts offered no real solution to a problem of health care of the magnitude that France had, pressed to improve and change the hospital situation. This reform effort was visible in Paris, for example, in at least three distinct ways: first, the improvement and enlargement of several old hospitals, especially the Hôtel-Dieu and the Charité; second, the creation of hospitals devoted to one specific and prevalent medical problem, such as the Hôpital du Midi, a convent in the Faubourg Saint Jacques which in 1784 became a hospital for venereal diseases; and third, the erection of new, smaller hospitals. Between 1775 and 1785 as many hospitals were founded in Paris as in the preceding 130 years, including the Clinique de Perfectionnement (1775), the Necker (1778), the Cochin (1780), the Maison de Santé (1781), and the Beaujon and the Midi (1784).[30]

In 1788, Tenon's classic report showed 28 hospitals in Paris containing 6,236 patients and 20 hospice-like places of care for 14,105 invalids.[31] There were several classes of hospitals. Those primarily for the sick, including the Santé, the Hôtel-Dieu, Incurables, and the Saint-Louis, were supervised by the Bureau of the Hôtel-Dieu, headed by the Archbishop of Paris. Hospitals for the aged and indigent were administered by the Bureau of the Hôpital-General, which consisted of the Bureau of the Hôtel-Dieu plus 18 laymen. Among this group of hospitals were the Bicêtre, the Salpêtrière, and the Pitié. The Grand Bureau des Pauvres operated two domiciliary hospitals, the Petites-Maisons for the aged and the Trinité for children.[32]

The challenge faced by the prerevolutionary reform movement can be better visualized through a brief survey of some of these Paris hospitals. Although the Hôtel-Dieu had existed since 829, it had burned in 1772 and been rebuilt. Located on the Ile de la Cité near the Petit Pont, this massive structure now had 1,400 beds but was still terribly overcrowded. In fact, as Tenon's report showed, conditions there were among the worst in Paris. The 200-bed Saint-Louis was built in the Faubourg du Temple in 1607 and its role as an ancient plague house was obvious.[33] The Incurables took its name from the condition of the patients it housed, while the Santé had a name that bore no resemblance to what its filthy walls contained.

Located across from the Jardin des Plantes were both the Pitié and the Salpêtrière. The former was an orphan asylum but it had benefited greatly from the influence of the Duc de la Rochefoucald-Liancourt's interest in hospital reform and vaccination. The latter, opened in 1656, was restricted to women and also served as a prison for beggars, paupers, and incurables. The equivalent institution for men was the Bicêtre. Among its patients were quite a few insane, who provided Philippe Pinel with ample resources for his famous studies on treatment of the insane.[34]

Those hospitals that lay outside the administrative reach of the Bureaus yielded somewhat more readily to reform efforts during the 1780s. The long, gray, stone buildings along the Boulevard des Invalides that comprised the Invalides complex were for the care of aged army veterans and were administered by the military medical service. The Invalides benefited from stricter regulations after 1781; and opposed to the Hôtel-Dieu, where one out of every three died, the mortality rate at the Invalides was only one in forty.[35] The Charité, located on the Rue St. Pères, also limited to males, was probably the best hospital in Paris and no more expensive than the Hôtel-Dieu. Founded in 1607 by the Brothers of Charity, it was famous for its lithotomists, and it was at the Charité that clinical teaching began under Desbois de Rochefort. A small success in the effort to specialize in diseases came with the conversion in 1784 of a convent in the Faubourg St. Jacques into the Hôpital du Midi for venereal patients. The Necker, on the Rue de Sèvres, was founded in 1778 with the specific intention of being a model medical facility. It was notable in that each of its 120 beds held only one person, and the cost was only 17 sous daily compared to 29 sous at the Hôtel-Dieu, 30 at the Charité, and 42 at the Incurables.[36]

As the prerevolutionary reform movement gathered momentum during the 1780s, the Paris hospitals came under a devastating attack from humanitarians, physicians, and scientists alike. For generations a typical complaint about hospitals had been the lack of fresh air in the wards, a condition based on the notion that fresh air carried evil humors. French hospitals were noted for their lack of ventilation and unsanitary bed curtains to prevent drafts. In 1784, the government of Louis XVI was finally persuaded to bear the full expense of installing huge bellows ventilators in a few of the big hospitals.[37]

The reformers were encouraged to begin exposing many other hospital evils and to clamor for their correction. Many observers noted how cold the hospitals were and charged that temperatures that commonly ranged between 3 and 5 degrees centigrade were a major cause of death.[38] Hospital gangrene (Vincent's bacillus) was shown to be endemic in every hospital. Highly contagious in filthy conditions, it invaded any break in the skin, covered the wound with a putrid, putty-colored coating, and brought the patient a violent fever, wracking pain, and eventually death.[39]

Reformers also complained about "priests coming in to give extreme unction to the dying, loudly and violently ringing bells, disturbing patients in need of sleep, and scaring the wits out of those who thought they might be dying."[40]

The multiplying number of crusaders for hospital reform in the 1780s produced scores of reports of investigations of hospitals in the larger towns and cities in France. The findings of conditions in these provincial hospitals were vividly described and summarized by the scientist Georges Cuvier: "The sufferings of hell can hardly surpass those of the poor wretches crowded on each other, crushed, burning with fever, incapable of stirring or breathing, sometimes having one or two dead people between them for hours."[41]

At the Bicêtre prison hospital in Paris, it was reported after investigation that there were three to four patients per bed, mixed indiscriminately by disease and sex. Jacques Beugnot, who called the hospital at the Conciergerie "the most horrifying in the world," said that "on the 45 to 50 beds along the two walls of the corridors, stagnating two by two, often three by three, are the unhappy victims of different diseases."[42] Lavoisier noted that the Saint Paul ward of the Hôtel-Dieu had 111 beds for 272 patients, and was also both a waiting room for the sick poor, and the passageway through which all supplies (including food) moved into the hospital and the soiled linen, human excreta, and corpses exited. At the same hospital, the insane were chained and whipped like animals. They were subjected to douches, cold baths, and antispasmodics regularly, and when highly agitated were given strong purgatives or profuse bleedings to weaken them. Sometimes they were suffocated.[43]

Responding to the growing outcry in 1786, the Royal Academy of Sciences named a special committee to investigate hospital conditions. All three members reported individually: a preliminary advice by the astronomer J.S. Bailly in late 1786, René Tenon's famous report in 1788, and Alphonse Leroy's analysis the following year.[44] At the same time, the classic studies of the English physician, John Howard, were being published and widely read in Europe. These contributed greatly to the suppression of typhus by showing its transmission under the prevailing conditions of filth and overcrowding in hospitals. Howard had visited Lyon and had praised the Charité hospital there (it was new), but he had nothing but condemnation for Lyon's Hôtel-Dieu, finding it "nasty and offensive, and two patients in many beds, but not one window open."[45] One can only speculate what Howard might have said had he seen the Hôtel-Dieu in Paris!

It was René Tenon who revealed conditions in Paris. His *Mémoires sur les hôpitaux de Paris* (1788), with its unforgettable descriptions of the Hôtel-Dieu, profoundly impressed Frenchmen. Tenon vividly described 1,220 beds, each holding four to six patients placed alternately head to foot. Only 426 beds held only one patient. Many so-called beds were but pallets or heaps of straw in vile condition. Vermin and filth abounded, as did hospital gangrene, septic fevers, and other infections; patients with acute contagious diseases lay haphazardly mixed with accident victims, dysentery sufferers, and patients with scrofula. Ventilation was still so poor that the physicians and surgeons, even the attendants, never entered the wards without a vinegar-dipped sponge held to their faces to thwart infection and neutralize the overpowering, ever-present stench. Recovery from surgery at the Hôtel-Dieu was rare. The man or woman who survived an operation usually perished from a disease contracted in the wards during convalescence.[46] After a comprehensive study, the chief army physician, Jean Coste, reported in 1789 that the Hôtel-Dieu had a mortality rate of one out of every three who entered. After hearing all of these reports (which were widely publicized by reformers), the Royal Society of Medicine threw its support to the reform movement. It launched a drive for hospital improvement calling for private beds, separate rooms, the separation of patients according to their ailments, and specialized hospitals for the insane and for unusual diseases. But it was very late, and the reform movement quickly lost momentum after the Bastille fell in July, 1789.[47]

Military hospitals in France had inevitably been involved in the hospital reform movement in the 1780s even though they were generally superior to civilian facilities. The Invalides in Paris with its 3,000 disabled or aged soldiers had been investigated by Tenon, but there was no criticism of it in his meticulous report of 1788. A five-year study (1782-87) of the seventy military and naval hospitals, conducted by the Academy of Sciences, had revealed a peacetime morality rate of only one in forty-two. In 1789, according to Coste who conducted a study of more than four months, it was still only one in forty.[48] But the military wards habitually maintained by the crown in civilian hospitals in peacetime were not included in either of these studies. The practice of placing sick soldiers in civilian hospitals was well established. In wartime, of course, the government took over many of them for military purposes, especially those near the front. Therefore it was often impossible to separate military and civilian medicine in eighteenth-century France. It was somewhat misleading to compare mortality rates of the military and civilian hospitals, but the difference was great enough to show that military hospitals gave the reformers little opportunity for a serious attack.

It was the growing crisis in government finances during the 1780s that began the disintegration of the superior military medical facilities. A harbinger of things to come in the military medical service was the short-lived Ordinance of January 1, 1780, which shut down the hospital ampitheaters for sake of economy. It relegated the five big teaching hospitals to auxiliary status. The reorganization proposed by the new inspector-general of prisons and hospitals, Jean Colombier, was aimed at creating hundreds of regimental hospitals.[49] The resulting outcry from the military medical service, the war commissioners, and the contractors, however, led to a reconsideration. The following spring (May 2, 1781), the teaching ampitheaters were reestablished, although Colombier persisted in advancing his ideas and plans for economy to an increasingly hard-pressed crown. Finally in 1788 the financial distress of the government was so acute that Colombier was told to draft new economy regulations and to recast the organization of French military medicine according to his own ideas.[50]

The resulting Ordinance of July 20, 1788, abolished all but eight naval and military hospitals and reserved these eight as "auxiliary depots" for sick and wounded who could not be cared for locally in civilian hospitals. It ended the teaching hospitals' ampitheaters. The hospitals that were to be created in each regiment were economy substitutes for the established military medical hospital system. The result was chaos. Suddenly responsible for their own sick and disabled, asked to arrange for hospital facilities in each regiment, and required to handle expenses for which there were no funds, the administrators of each corps found the task impossible. The ordinance was impractical even if funds had been available; frequent troop movements would have negated contracts between the local hospitals and army authorities and required their renegotiation in each new locality.[51]

Thus the great hospital reform movement prior to 1789, along with the accompanying efforts to improve the practice of medicine and the quality o health care in general, came face to face with the hard political and economic realities of the summer of 1789. In the ensuing turmoil, further reform of civilian medicine was lost in the momentous events of the day. The one area of acceptable medical care, the military medical service, was crippled and its patients referred to the amply demonstrated inadequacy of civilian hospitals. The abolition of the teaching ampitheaters was disastrous as the Revolutionary armies were to discover when war came and the shortage of adequate hospitals and trained medical men was painfully evident. When the Revolution broke, the timing was of critical importance for the future of French medicine. The evils of its civilian aspects had been laid bare by reformers for all to see; the military medical system was torn by internal dissension and was trying to reorganize itself—but under adverse financial circumstances and according to an ill-conceived plan.

NOTES

1. Albert Mathiez, "La mobilisation des savants en l'an II, " *Revue de Paris* 24: 544; J. J. A. Laboulbène, Histoire du journalisme médicale, 1679—1880," *Gazette des hôpitaux civils et militaires* 53: 1057, 1065, 1073, 1088—89.

2. Beatrice F. Hyslop, *Guide to the General Cahiers of 1789* (New York, 1936), passim.; Beatrice F. Hyslop, "Les cahiers de doléances de 1789," *Annales historique de la Révolution française* 27: 115—23.

3. Rosen, "Hospitals, Medical Care and Social Policy," *Bull. Hist. Med.* 30: 124—26.

4. *Edit du roi, portant création d'Offices de Conseillers de Sa Majesté, Médecins et Chirurgiens Inspecteurs Généraux, et Majors à la suite des armées, dans tous les Hôpitaux, Villes Frontières, et ancien Régiments. Donné à Versailles, au mois de janvier 1708* (Paris, 1708), pp.1—4.

5. *Edit du Roy, portant suppression des charges de Médecins et de Chirurgiens, créés par edit du mois de janvier 1708. Donné à Paris, au mois de juin 1716* (Paris, 1716), pp.1—4.

6. Cilleuls, "Les médecins," *Revue hist. de l'armée* 6: 10; *Dict. encyclopédique sci. méd.*, 2d ser., 8: 81—83.

7. Uniform regulations included *Formules de pharmacie pour les hôpitaux militaires du Roy* (Paris, 1747) and the basic rules which were frequently amended but remained the heart of the 1788 edition of *Formules de médicaments rédigées dans la Conseil de Santé des hôpitaux militaires par ordre du Conseil de guerre* (Paris, 1788).

8. "Since soldiers had a repugnance for Keyser's mercury pills for syphilis and would spit them out after the physicians had departed, Choiseul as early as 1767 had issued orders that the physicians stay long enough to be sure the pills went down." McCloy, *Government Assistance*, p.166. See also Garrison, *Notes*, p.156.

9. Rieux and Hassenforder, *Histoire*, p.9; George Fischer, "Surgery One Hundred Years Ago," *Journal of the American Medical Association* 29: 588.

10. Ambroise Paré, *La manière de traicter les playes faictes tant par hacquebutes, que par flèches; et les accidentz d'icelles, comme fractures et caries des os, gangrène et mortification; avec les pourtraictz des instrumentz nécessaires pour leur curation. Et le méthode de curer les combustions principalement faicts par la pouldre à canon* (Paris, 1552); Carlos d'Eschevannes, *La vie d'Ambroise Paré, père de la chirurgie, 1510–1590* (Paris, 1930), passim; *Dict. encyclopédique sci. méd.*, 2d ser., 21: 127.

11. Quoted in Garrison, *Notes*, p.152.

12. Briot, *Chirurgie militaire*, pp.80–81, 388.

13. Short of a visit to the Museum Val-de-Grâce in Paris, a good view of the "surgical arsenal" produced by the mid-century wars may be found in Sauveur François Morand, *Catalogue des pièces d'anatomie, instrumens, machines, &c. qui composent l'arsenal de chirurgie* (Paris, 1759) and in Denis Diderot, *Encyclopédie des sciences: Chirurgie* (Paris, 1780), Plate XXI, Fig. 1.

14. Jean Louis Petit (1674–1750) of Paris, specialist in aneurisms and bones: Petit dossier, carton 212, Val-de-Grâce. A number of Petit's devices are shown in his *Treatise on the Diseases of the Bones* (London, 1726), passim.

15. Diderot, *Chirurgie*, Plate XVIII, Fig. 1 (Petit's screw tourniquet), Plate X, Fig. 7 (Desault's forceps), Plate X, Fig. 9 (Perret's dressing forceps and Petit's artery forceps); McCloy, *French Inventions*, pp.161–62; Thompson, *Surgical Instruments*, pp.67–68, 85. Jean Jacques Perret (1730–84) of Béziers became the top Paris manufacturer of surgical instruments, especially well known for his dressing forceps and cataract knives, *Nouvelle biographie* 39: 642. Pierre Joseph Desault (1744–95) rose from the son of a poor farmer to surgeon-in-chief of the Hôtel Dieu in Paris (1785), where he established a surgical clinic: Desault dossier, carton 206, Val-de-Grâce. See also *Dict. encyclopédique sci. méd.*, 1st ser., 28: 272.

16. Ravaton, a fine military surgeon, began two-flap amputations. See descriptions and illustrations of the "tin boot" in Hugues Ravaton, *Chirurgie d'armée* (Paris, 1768) and in Diderot, *Chirurgie*, Plate IV, Fig. 3. Antoine Louis (1723–92) of Metz, permanent secretary of the Royal Academy of Surgery from 1744, regimental surgeon-major of the Army of the Rhine, 1760: Carton 112, Arch. hist. Service de Santé, and Louis dossier, carton 209/1, Val-de-Grâce. Pierre François Percy (1754–1825) of Montagney in Haute-Saône, famous military surgeon of the Revolutionary and Napoleonic wars and a Baron of the Empire: Percy dossier, carton 211 bis, Val-de-Grâce. See also Charles Laurent, *Histoire de la vie et des ouvrages de P. F. Percy, composées sur les manuscrits originaux* (Versailles, 1827). A *tribulcon* (Percy's divided forceps), one part a probe to be inserted into a wound first, then the other blade inserted to lock on and

extract by squeezing on the bullet, is detailed in Diderot, *Chirurgie*, Plate IX, Fig. 4.

17. Ordinance of August 4, 1772, in carton 1, Arch. hist. Service de Santé; *Dict. encyclopédique sci. méd.*, 2d ser., 7: 86; Fischer, "Surgery," *Jour. Am. Med. Assn.* 29: 540.

18. Quoted in Charles L. Heizmann, "Military Sanitation in the Sixteenth, Seventeenth, and Eighteenth Centuries," *Annals of Medical History* 1: 298–99. Regulations required the mobile hospital to remain one league distant from the action. Jacques Bagieu (c.1700–57), a long-time surgeon of the Royal Guards, *Dict. encyclopédique sci. méd.*, 1st ser., 8: 90.

19. *Réglement fait par ordre du roi, pour établir dans les Hôpitaux militaires de Strasbourg, Metz, et Lille, des ampithéâtres destinés à former en médecine, chirurgie, et pharmacie, des Officiers de santé pour le service des Hôpitaux militaires du royaume et des armées. Du 22 septembre 1775* (Paris, 1775), carton 1 (Laws and Decrees), Arch. hist. Service de Santé. See also *Dict. encyclopédique sci. méd.*, 2d ser., 8: 84–85.

20. Cilleuls, "Chirurgiens militaires de l'ancien régime," *Revue hist. de l'armée* 6: 11; Augustin Cabanès, *Chirurgiens et blessés à travers l'histoire* (Paris, 1918), p.300.

21. M. Bottet, "Le passé: le service de santé et les commissaires des guerres," *Caducée* 5: 151.

22. *Ordonnance Royale du 2 mai 1781 portant règlement sur la constitution et l'administration générale des hôpitaux militaires* (Versailles, 1781): Carton 1, Arch. hist. Service de Santé. Ordinances of 1772, 1777, and 1781 are also in *Dict. encyclopédique sci. méd.*, 2d ser., 8: 86–88.

23. Jean François Coste (1741–1819) of Bugey (Ain), son of a physician, first physician of Rochambeau's army in America (1780–83). Chief navy physician (1783), chief of health service of northern provinces (1784), then first physician of the army camps. Recalled to Versailles in 1789, elected mayor in 1790. He served as a military physician during the wars of the Revolution and Empire: Coste dossier, carton 205/1, Val-de-Grâce. Pierre Coze (1754–1822) of Ambleteuse (Pas-de-Calais): Coze dossier, carton 205/1, ibid.; Charles Louis Dumas (1765–1813) of Lyon: Dumas dossier, carton 206/1, ibid.; Claude Antoine Lombard (1741–1811) of Dôle, in 1790 surgeon-in-chief of civil and military hospitals: Lombard dossier, carton 209/1, ibid.; Nicolas Saucerotte (1741–1814): Saucerotte dossier, carton 209/1, ibid.; Joseph Adam Lorentz (1734–1801), veteran of the Seven Years War and physician-in-chief of the Army of the Rhine in 1792: Lorentz dossier, carton 209/1, ibid.; Pierre Christophe Gorcy (1758–1826) of Pont-à-Mousson: Gorcy dossier, carton 14, Arch. hist. Service de Santé; Jean François Thomassin (1750– ?) of Rochefort: Thomassin dossier, cartons 22 and 28, ibid.; Nicolas Heurteloup (1750–1819), Acquisitions françaises, 21a, pp.27–30,

Archives nationales, Paris. See above for biographical note on Percy.

24. Raphael Bienvenu Sabatier (1732–1811) of Paris, son of a St. Côme surgeon, member of the Academy of Sciences in 1773 and, after Louis, permanent secretary of the Academy of Surgery (1792–1811), consulting physician of the Army of the North (1792), inspector-general of health of the armies and professor of practical medicine (1795) at the Paris Ecole de Santé: Sabatier dossier, carton 213, Val-de-Grâce. Pierre Sue (1739–1816) of Paris, professor of therapeutics in the School of Surgery (1790), interim secretary of the Academy of Surgery (1792), chief physician of the army of the Russian campaign of 1812, Reports of the Corps de Santé, carton 22, Arch. hist. Service de Santé. See above for biographical notes on Corvisart, Desault, and Louis.

25. McCloy, *Government Assistance*, pp.416–17.

26. *Arch. parl.* 22: 388. Pichault de la Martinière (1696–1783), First Surgeon to Louis XV and Louis XVI, *Dict. encyclopédique sci. méd.*, 2d ser., 5: 165.

27. The Society of Medicine's contest dealt with tetanus: *Société de Médecine, Projet d'instruction sur une maladie convulsive, fréquente dans les colonies de l'Amerique connue sous le nom de Tetanos* (Paris, 1786). In 1789, the Academy of Surgery's award was offered for a study of surgical instruments. See Briot, *Chirurgie militaire*, pp.36–37; Smeaton, *Fourcroy*, p.2; and Boutry, "La médecine," *Chron. méd.* 11: 742.

28. Ackernecht, *Paris Hospital*, p.16.

29. Boutry, "La médecine," *Chron. méd.* 11: 740; McCloy, *Government Assistance*, p.452; Laignel-Lavastine, *Histoire générale* 3: 692.

30. Ackernecht, *Paris Hospital*, pp.17–21.

31. René Tenon, *Mémoires sur les hôpitaux de Paris* (Paris, 1788).

32. Rosen, "Hospitals, Medical Care and Social Policy," *Bull. Hist. Med.* 30: 131–32.

33. Ackernecht, *Paris Hospital*, pp.19–21.

34. Ibid.

35. Report dossier, folio A, carton 205, Val-de-Grâce.

36. Laignel-Lavastine, *Histoire générale* 3: 692; McCloy, *Government Assistance*, p.452; Boutry, "La médecine," *Chron. méd.* 11: 740.

37. Stephen Hales invented this method of artificial ventilation in 1743, using animal power to operate the huge bellows: McCloy, *French Inventions*, p.120.

38. Ackernecht, *Paris Hospital*, p.19.

39. Garrison, *Notes*, p.155; Edmond Delorme, *War Surgery* (London, 1915), pp.116–17.

40. Boutry, "La médecine," *Chron. méd.* 11: 738.

41. Quoted in Gershoy, *Despotism to Revolution*, p.293. Georges Leopold Cuvier (1769–1832) of Montbèliard, distinguished French physicist, naturalist and botanist, *Dict. encyclopédique sci. méd.*, 1st ser.,

24: 452—56. Also see William Coleman, *Georges Cuvier, Zoologist: A Study in the History of Evolution Theory* (Cambridge, Mass., 1964).

42. Quoted in Laignel-Lavastine, *Histoire générale* 3: 699. Comte Jacques Claude Beugnot (1761—1835) of Aube, deputy from Aube to the Legislative Assembly, opponent of Marat, arrested in 1793 and imprisoned, released after the events of 9 Thermidor, *Nouvelle biographie*, 5: 859—61.

43. Tenon, *Mémoires*, passim; McKie, *Lavoisier*, p.202.

44. Jean Sylvain Bailly (1736—93) of Paris, president of the National Assembly after the Tennis Court meeting and Mayor of Paris after the fall of the Bastille. He lost popularity after the Champ de Mars and was executed. René Tenon (1724—1816) of Scepeaux near Joigny, son of a physician, served in Flanders as a surgeon first-class in 1744, then was first surgeon at the Salpêtrière. Professor of pathology in the School of Surgery in Paris in 1785, member of the Legislative Assembly from Seine-et-Oise. He retired to Massey in 1793, returned to Paris after 9 Thermidor. *Dict. encyclopédique sci. méd.*, 3d ser., 16: 393. Alphonse Vincent Leroy (1742—1816) of Paris, member of the Academy of Sciences and author of *Précis d'un ouvrage sur les hôpitaux* (Paris, 1789), ibid., 2d ser., 2: 199.

45. John Howard, *An Account of the Principal Lazarettos in Europe* (Warrington, Engl., 1789), p.52. The Charité in Lyon was new, having been torn down in 1783 and rebuilt completely by 1786. See also A. Camelin, "Lyon et médecine militaire," *Revue hist. de l'armée* 16: 88.

46. Tenon, *Mémoires*, passim.

47. Coste dossier, folio A, carton 205/1, Val-de-Grâce.

48. Ibid.

49. Rieux and Hassenforder, *Histoire*, pp.10—12. Jean Colombier (1736—89) of Toul, product of the military hospital at Metz and a regimental surgeon-major until 1780 when he became inspector-general of the prisons and hospitals of France. He died a few months after securing approval of his draft of the Ordinance of July 20, 1788. *Dict. encyclopédique sci. méd.*, 1st ser., 19: 74.

50. *Ordonnance Royale du 2 mai 1781*, carton 1 (Laws and Decrees) Arch. hist. Service de Santé.

51. *Ordonnance Royale de 20 juillet 1788*. Ibid.

Chapter Three

MEDICAL MEN AND
THE POLITICAL REVOLUTION, 1789-1792

Early in 1789 students flocked to Paris just as they had done in previous years. Nearly one thousand surgical students alone had come to study at the School of Surgery or to follow the teaching of Desault at the Hôtel-Dieu, or of Corvisart at the Charité, or of Sabatier at the Invalides.[1] Students in every stage of medical training gravitated to the capital because cadavers were easily obtained there and were especially plentiful after the freezing winter of 1788—89. Because Paris symbolized opportunity for middle-class Frenchmen, eager young aspirants to the medical profession tolerated the Spartan student life. One could always make a little money by tutoring, by carrying out research and by ghostwriting for wealthy men, or by finding a low-paying assistantship in one of the schools or hospitals.[2]

Opportunity lay in securing any position in the Paris medical world, usually through a patron's influence. Some students had been in Paris for years seeking a place. One such was a young physician of Thonon, Dessaix, who came to visit the Paris hospitals in 1786, attached himself to the celebrated Berthollet, but still found all avenues of advancement closed.[3] Another was Alexis Boyer, who had risen from an Uzerches farm to become a Paris master barber's boy. He grubbed an existence by tutoring beginners at the School of Surgery and was acquiring what training he could in 1789 by joining the crowd that surged around Desault as he made his rounds at the Hôtel-Dieu. In the same swarm of students was Antoine Dubois from Gramat, also frustrated and poor. In March, 1789, Desault finally nominated both Boyer and Dubois for a second subassistantship in surgery under Sabatier at the Invalides. There were 38 candidates for the place. Jean Larrey, the nominee of Antoine Louis, headed the list. What happened on the day of selection was all too common. The Count de Puységur, Minister of War, struck Larrey's name, substituted that of his own protégé, and awarded the place to him.[4]

Young men like these eager but rejected candidates, already aware of the glaring defects in medical education, yet earnestly pursuing what training they could find, found the inequities of the Old Regime increasingly intolerable. From students who knew physical hardships and bitter disappointments, revolutionaries were made; they became "searching critics imbued with attitudes that were not to be reconciled with the *status quo*."[5] Many of their elders in the medical profession stimulated the increasingly radical attitudes of the younger generation. Among the established Paris physicians who were clever agitators were Peter J. G. Cabanis, an ardent liberal and a friend of Mirabeau, and Joseph Guillotin, whose *Pétition des Citoyens domiciliés à Paris* (December 8, 1788) gained for him an early notoriety. At the Lycée de la Rue Valois, Antoine Fourcroy taught chemistry brilliantly, but the Paris Faculty of Medicine still denied him the *docteur regent*; between lectures in the spring of 1789, he was demanding freedom of the press and laboring with some four hundred others of the Third Estate to prepare the Paris *cahiers* for the Estates-General that had been summoned.[6]

In that august body, which assembled at Versailles on May 5, 1789, there appeared a number of liberal physicians. Brillat-Savarin was sent to represent the Third Estate of Ain, and from an obscure practice in the Vendée came Jean Gallot, a Protestant.[7] J. B. Salle, a house physician at Nancy, entered the Estates-General along with Pierre Bouisson, deputy from the Sénéchaussée of Agen.[8] Joining them was none other than Joseph Guillotin, representing Paris. In every case, the 17 physicians in the Estates-General (all of whom carried over into the National Assembly) were notable not for their medical achievements but for their political liberalism.[9]

The Réveillon riots of late April, 1789, furnished students and teachers with both medical opportunity and some political excitement. Beginning with the plundering of the home of Réveillon, a wealthy Paris wallpaper manufacturer, the affair became a bloody encounter between the mob and regular troops.[10] Its aftermath afforded many their first look at wounds freshly made by military firearms. Desault gathered his students, teaching them the use of Paré's emollients for gunshot wounds, forbidding bleeding and extensive wound excision, and demonstrating to Boyer, Dubois, Larrey, and others how to cut away bruised and ragged wound edges and unite them with sutures. Unfortunately for many of those wounded in the Réveillon fracas, Desault insisted that amputation was a last resort. Consequently, Larrey observed, Desault lost most of these patients to tetanus.[11]

Bloodshed and the air of political crisis in Paris having already interfered with medical training, teachers and students alike became more active politically. They were attracted by talk of a Paris militia, an idea which grew increasingly popular after the Paris electors of the deputation to the Estates-General met on the night of July 4 to discuss it. The night of July 13 saw well-organized bands of medical, surgical, and law students roaming the streets of Paris in search of arms. There were nearly five hundred surgical students, including Larrey, who marched around all night, arousing the sections. The old veterans at Sabatier's Hôtel des Invalides sympathized with the revolutionaries, and the veterinarian Lafosse was one of the first to carry weapons to the mob from the hospital magazine.[12]

The revolutionary group at the Paris City Hall on July 14 included 154 lawyers, 26 merchants, 13 physicians and surgeons, 5 deputies including Guillotin, and 2 members of the Academy of Sciences, Bailly and Fourcroy.[13] In the mob that they directed toward the Bastille were Lafosse, the physician Dessaix, and surgeons Larrey, Boyer, and Dubois. The view expressed by Paul Triaire, that these students were not revolutionaries but just young, excited enthusiasts, is not supported by the evidence. They had organized during the previous night, armed themselves, and participated actively in storming the Bastille. They were mature enough by the standards of the eighteenth century: Larrey was 23 years old, Dessaix 25, Lafosse about 30, Boyer 32, and Dubois 33. Both Dessaix and Larrey spoke of the "ardor" with which they participated in the revolutionary events of July 14, 1789. Larrey wrote: "I headed a group of 1,500 young people and we were the first to march against the tyrants."[14]

Politically active physicians and surgeons could be found with a high degree of consistency in almost any cross-section of the Revolution. Most embraced its principles heartily. In his study of the Jacobins, Professor Crane Brinton noted how extremely common during the Revolution was "that familiar figure, the radical physician."[15] After the Bastille, medical men appeared in the Phrygian bonnet, wearing the revolutionary cockade and the short revolutionary vest, having discarded their knee breeches, gold-lace-trimmed coats, wigs, and earrings. High top shoes, trousers, and plain short coat marked the return of physicians to simple bourgeois dress. Many appeared in the new uniform of the National Guard, parading in the public celebrations.[16]

Members of the medical profession also turned up in elective offices of their communes, districts, departments, and even in the national assemblies. The surgeon Jacques Cassanyes, who wrote that he "was counted and recognized as a patriot in 1789," was mayor of Canet, founder of its National Guard, a director of the district of Perpignan, a deputy to the Convention, and a representative on mission during the Jacobin régime.[17] The apothecaries Opoix and Campmartin became mayors of Provins (Seine-et-Marne) and St. Girons (Ariège), respectively. The army physician J. F. Coste was recalled to Versailles and served as mayor from February 8, 1790, to January 7, 1792. The physician Guillemardet became mayor of Autun (Saône-et-Loire), and Prunelle de Lière was elected mayor of Grénoble early in 1791. Two physicians who were elected justices of the peace, Pierre Duhem of Lille and Beauvais de Préau of Paris, were rabid revolutionaries.[18] The district administrator of Mans was the surgeon Levasseur, and physicians tapped as departmental administrators included Jard-Panvillier (Deux Sèvres), Lacoste (Dordogne), Carrère (Perpignan), and Valdruche (Haute-Marne).[19] After July, 1789, Fourcroy practiced medicine and helped J. S. Bailly, astronomer-mayor of Paris, govern the city until the 1790 Commune was formed. Although Fourcroy dropped out, the Paris Commune of 131 men still included 6 physicians. After the National Assembly expired in September, 1791, Brillat-Savarin returned to Ain as president of the civil court and mayor of Belley, Gallot was named administrator in the Vendée, and Salle became a member of the directory of the Meurthe.[20]

In these early years of the Revolution, physicians were almost invariably leaders in forming local political clubs. The Society of Friends of the Rights of Man and the Citizen (which met at the Convent of the Cordeliers) was founded in Paris in the summer of 1790 by the physician Saintex, the printer Momoro, and the engineer Duforny.[21] Having lingered in Paris for a year after helping to take the Bastille, Dessaix returned to practice in his native Savoy and fell in with his radical compatriot, the physician François Doppet. They founded at Chambéry the Société de propaganda des Alpes in September, 1790, and then moved to Thonon to form the Club des patriotes étrangers. The founders of Jacobin clubs were usually local men of position and substance, lawyers, physicians, and businessmen, whether in the cities like Bordeaux or in tiny villages like Artonne.[22]

In the small town of Bergerac (Dordogne) the physician Boissière was one of five Jacobin leaders, and Bigourdan held a similar distinction in the tiny Gascon village of Fleurance. The physician Desbart was one of seven Jacobin founders in Gerberay in the Oise. At Moulins, two physicians and an apothecary served terms as president of the local Jacobin group. One of the top three Jacobins at Mayence was the physician Wedekind. Montrolle was among six leaders at Nancy while "the brothers Bonac, one a lawyer and the other a physician and leading men in the little town of Pellagrue (Gironde), were the very life of the local club, even in the Terror."[23]

At Limoges and Toulouse, physicians were very much evident in the Jacobin leadership, and both clubs had active committees of health. The Limoges committee of physicians, surgeons, and apothecaries gave free medical treatment to the poor at club expense. The Toulouse group campaigned against the bad nursing and poor sanitary conditions in the local hospitals. The interest taken by Jacobin clubs in general in the realm of public hygiene attests to the almost universal presence of medical men in their membership and, as Brinton observed, constitutes "one of the very definitely modern things" about these clubs.[24] On the other hand, their activity of political surveillance is illustrated by the Bacqueville club's rejection of the surgeon Sellier "because he consorted with priests, though Sellier claimed he was just trying to 'convert' them. Le Pley, another surgeon, was kept on the roll after he promised to make only brief and purely professional calls on 'aristocrats'."[25]

By the spring of 1791, the efforts of the National Assembly to stabilize the Revolution with a constitutional monarchy began to encounter resistance. Republican ideas were spreading through the fast-growing Jacobin clubs. When Pope Pius VI formally condemned all of the principles of the Revolution, towns, villages, and families split violently, and Frenchmen in 1791 seemed forced to choose between Catholicism and the Revolution. Because of this bitter religious controversy and his own aversion to constitutional limitations, Louis XVI determined to flee from France. His party got as far as Varennes in mid June before being recognized and returned to Paris. Radical clubs and newspapers called loudly for a republic, and the sullen crowds revealed a deep hostility to the suspect king. The gathering of republicans at the Champ de Mars on the second anniversary of the fall of the Bastille had to be forcibly dispersed by Paris authorities. Over forty republicans were killed.[26]

The National Assembly finally promulgated the Constitution of 1791 in September. The king accepted it, and a new assembly, the Legislative, convened on October 1. Twenty-eight deputies were listed as physicians. None sat on the Right. Only a few occupied the Center. Among the latter were Jard-Panvillier from Deux-Sèvres, Plaichard-Choltière from Mayenne, Masuyer from Saône-et-Loire, René Tenon from Seine-et-Oise, and Pierre Broussonnet from Paris.[27] The great majority of medical men were on the Left. In addition to the rabid Jacobin Beauvais de Préau from Paris, there were, for example, the violent Pierre Duhem from Lille, Valdruche from the Haute-Marne, Lacoste and Taillefer from Dordogne, Siblot from the Haute-Saône, the radical Bô from Aveyron, Baudot from Saône-et-Loire, and Clédel from Lot.[28]

Of this new legislative body of 745 representatives, about one-third (the

Right) supported the constitutional monarchy. The majority, or Center, was not committed, but the Left was determined to discredit the king and establish a republic. The radical Left wanted a "war of peoples against kings," while those on the Right, who wanted to preserve the monarchy, came to see in war a hope that Louis XVI could regain his power.

With both the Left and the Right of the Legislative Assembly desiring hostilities for different reasons, France declared war on Austria and Prussia on April 20, 1792. But military reverses on the frontier, fear of invasion, defections to the enemy, bread shortages, rising prices, and suspicions of treachery by the crown all heightened popular nationalistic and revolutionary feelings. An armed mob stormed into the Tuileries on August 10, 1792. They massacred the Swiss Guard, imprisoned the royal family, and ended the short-lived constitutional monarchy.[29]

The Constitution of 1791 was also dead, and the Legislative Assembly had no choice but to call for new elections. Universal manhood suffrage was authorized for the selection of a National Convention to create a republic. Meanwhile, Longwy and Verdun fell to the advancing enemy, and Lafayette fled to Austria. Finally General Dumouriez's victory at Valmy on September 20 forced the Prussians to retire into winter quarters. On September 22 the Convention assembled, immediately concerned with a new constitution, the war, and the trial of Louis XVI for treason.[30]

All of these events involved the radical physician. P. J. G. Cabanis was a member of the Revolutionary Tribunal for a while, and one of the most ferocious judges of this period was the lithotomist J. Souberbielle. One of the heroes of the arrest of the King at Varennes was a surgeon, Jean Mangin, who was rewarded by the Convention with a position in the military hospital at Metz. At the Champ de Mars on July 14, 1791, Larrey and his colleagues wheelbarrowed dirt and stones for barricades and later retired to the Invalides and bandaged wounded men. After Bailly's arrest, the epidemiologist N. Chambon de Montaux served in 1792 as moderate mayor of Paris. Dessaix, chased from Savoy for his Jacobin activities, returned to Paris and appeared as captain of a detachment which helped to massacre the Swiss Guards at the Tuileries on August 10. The radical Beauvais de Préau, deputy from Paris to the Legislative Assembly, was the physician in the deputation that visited Louis XVI after August 10 to tell him of his deposition.[31]

As the Revolution moved to the left, radical physicians were even more in evidence. There were 17 medical men in the National Assembly, 28 in the Legislative Assembly of 1791 (3.7 percent), and 49 in the National Convention of September, 1792 (6 percent). There were signs, however, that the Convention was too radical for some. J. B. Salle, a radical in the

National Assembly of 1790, was aligned with the Girondin leadership of the Convention but was being forced further to the right by the Jacobins. One who now supported Louis XVI openly and took his seat with the Right was Grénoble's mayor, the physician Prunelle de Lière. Broussonnet, who had been in the Legislative Assembly's Center, moved over to the Right in the National Convention and, when the king's trial opened, fled to Spain. Both De Lière and J. B. Salle voted against the execution of Louis XVI.[32]

There were three physicians elected to the National Convention who had occupied the Legislative Assembly's Center with Broussonnet: Masuyer, Plaichard-Choltière, and Jard-Panvillier. All three again aligned themselves with the Center (Plain). The number of physicians here was more than doubled, however, by new deputies coming in. The apothecary Opoix, deputy of Seine-et-Marne, took his seat with the Plain. Pierre Bodin, a surgeon at Limeray (Indre-et-Loire), the physician Jean Defrance (Seine-et-Marne), and a physician from Vierzat (Creuse), Jean Baraillon, were partisans of "liberty without license" in the moderate middle of the Convention. All of the medical men of the Right and Center of the National Convention including J. B. Salle and de Lière voted against the death of the king.[33]

An increased number of medical men had also strengthened the Convention's Left (the Mountain). Radicals who had been in the Legislative Assembly, such as Duhem, De Préau, Baudot, Bô, Clédel, Lacoste, Taillefer, Siblot, and Valdruche, were elected to the Convention, and they took their seats again on the Left. Bouisson, formerly in the National Assembly, unlike Salle remained a radical in the Convention. Joining the Mountain were three other physicians, Jean Paul Marat of Paris, Ferdinand Guillemardet (Seine-et-Loire), and François Lanthenas (Rhône-et-Loire). Indicative of the entries from the lower social and economic ranks of the middle class were the apothecary Pierre Campmartin of Saint Girons (Arriège), the surgeon Jacques Cassanyes (Perpignan), and a surgeon-midwife (*accoucheur*) representing the Sarthe, René Levasseur.[34] To a man, these radical republicans of the medical profession voted death for Louis XVI.

Although the Legislative Assembly's 28 medical men had included one physician of reputation, Jacques René Tenon, the Convention's medical contingent of 49 contained not one of a similar reputation. The larger number of apothecaries and surgeons was indicative of the trend wherein control of the Revolution was passing from the upper bourgeoisie to the lower middle class. In his *French Revolution*, Thompson demonstrated this in another way by a comparison of the personnel of the Paris

Communes. Lawyers declined in numbers from 44 in the 1790 Commune of 131 members (33 percent) to 31 in the 1792 Commune of 201 members (15 percent), while merchant-tradesmen rose in number from 42 (32 percent) to 104 (50 percent), and artists from 12 (9 percent) to 34 (17 percent). There were 6 physicians in the 1790 Commune (4.6 percent), 5 physicians in the 1791 Commune (3.7 percent), and only 4 in the 1792 Commune (2 percent).[35]

"Remarkably," wrote the French historian Georges Pouchet, "one cannot find a single man of science among the emigrés, not even from Lyon, Toulon, the Vendée. All had embraced the cause of the Revolution."[36] This sweeping claim is quite false. Donald Greer produced a statistical study of this emigration which noted 587 physicians and surgeons among 2,683 middle-class emigrés. They were almost equally divided: 294 physicians and 292 surgeons. In the lower middle class, Greer found 68 apothecaries, 50 druggists, and 15 pharmacists who fled France but only 17 midwives, 7 nurses, and 3 dentists. There does not appear to have been a genuine barber-surgeon among the 173 classified as emigrés.[37]

In view of the family position occupied by these emigré physicians and surgeons attached to the nobility, their exit with noble families was not surprising. Typical of them was the physician to Monsieur (Louis XVIII), Lefebvre Saint-Ildefont, who emigrated with his royal patron to Holland, Germany, and Italy. A second wave of emigration included physicians such as P. Vitet and Joseph Carrère, whose revolutionary zeal had cooled by 1792, and Pierre Broussonnet, appalled by the prospect of trying the king, who fled from the Legislative Assembly to Spain in September, 1792. Another tide of emigration during the Terror included Anthelme Brillat-Savarin, probably a victim of a professional vendetta since he was denounced by a Belley apothecary, Bonnet, and another local physician, Carrier.[38]

It may be said that the vast majority of men in the medical profession stayed with the Revolution, but their fortunes varied widely. A few were men ennobled and loaded with pensions like Pierre Poissonier, the inspector-general of naval hospitals, who was imprisoned in the Saint Lazare until released to die in poverty; while Louis Le Monnier, physician to both Louis XV and Louis XVI, remained at the Tuileries until he was confined to the Luxembourg on August 10, 1792, and was later released to vegetate in a poor mediocrity and raise herbs. The physician of the Louvre and the Bastille, Jacques Philibert Read, stayed to become First Physician to the Constitutional Guard of Louis XVI in 1791 and then ended his career in the military hospital at Saint Quentin in a poorly paid and obscure position.[39]

On the other hand, Sabatier's career at the Invalides remained peaceful and sedentary. He was undisturbed by the Revolution and, as Percy once said, "on his way to fame, Sabatier encountered only admirers."[40] Philippe Pinel reigned at the Bicêtre in 1792, after having gained stature for advancing the science of psychiatry through his report to the National Assembly (1791) on the treatment of the insane. Although sometimes harassed, Desault and Pelletan remained at the Hôtel-Dieu. In the cluster of students there during 1790–92 were Jean Larrey, François Ribes, Jean Péborde, Bernard Bérot, and Xavier Bichat, the founder of the science of histology.[41] The latter, after he had fled from Lyon to Paris, studied under Corvisart, the founder of clinical medicine, who was still at the Charité. Corvisart was followed by such students as Rene Laënnec, the inventor of the stethoscope (1819), and Pierre Bretonneau, the discoverer of diphtheria (1826).[42] Still at the School of Surgery in Paris were Pierre Sue and Desault's friend François Chopart. The latter was pioneering surgery of the urinary tract and developing a foot amputation technique (1792) that still bears his name.[43]

Fourcroy and François Doublet moved into leadership of the Society of Medicine, turning out a great volume of reports on such subjects as "cosmetics, cough-cures, remedies for toothache, pomades, cast-iron water taps, fountains for purifying water, and machines for preparing vapor baths."[44] Nicolas Dubois de Chémant invented improved false teeth, and Antoine Louis and Joseph Guillotin collaborated on the invention of the "louisette" or, as it became known, the guillotine. Berthollet left medical practice for chemical research, publishing (1791) his *Elemens de l'art de teinture* on chlorine bleaching.[45] Grasset de Saint-Saveur invented a hammock for transporting wounded soldiers, and Jean Larrey received a gold medal and 100 livres in 1791 for his new suture needles.[46] Pierre Percy, who had invented a bullet extractor in 1790, published early in 1792 the most famous manual of military surgery of the period, *Manuel du chirurgien d'armée*. A textile designer from Lyon, Philippe de Lasalle, invented an adjustable hospital bed in 1791, and at the College of Surgery in Paris, Oudet began the production of artificial limbs in 1792.[47]

From a professional standpoint, French medical men generally found that their routine was little changed during the early years of the Revolution. The top physicians and surgeons of the big hospitals and of military medicine remained at their posts, busy with their work. Teaching, writing, invention, and practical medicine continued to flourish in a revolutionary climate that was favorable to "science." Politically, things were different. A phenomenon of the Revolution was the appearance of radical physicians in positions of top political leadership. Active in local, provincial, and national assemblies, these men represented a completely new influence in French political life. The vast majority of them were medical unknowns before the Revolution; their qualifications for important offices rested almost solely upon their liberal political views. When the national assemblies began dismantling the Old Regime, the medical profession was deeply involved and well represented.

NOTES

1. Smeaton, *Fourcroy*, p.1.

2. Cabanès, *Médecins amateurs*, p.328.

3. "Le Docteur-Général Dessaix," *Chron. méd.* 16: 700.

4. André Soubiran, *Le baron Larrey, chirurgien de Napoléon* (Paris, 1967), p.45; *Dict. encyclopédique sci. méd.*, 1st ser., 10: 424; 30: 605.

5. Gershoy, *From Despotism to Revolution*, p.276.

6. P. J. G. Cabanis, *On the Degree of Certainty in Medicine* (Philadelphia, 1828), pp.6—18; Ackernecht, *Paris Hospital*, pp.3—8. Joseph Ignace Guillotin (1738—1814) of Saintes (Charenté-Inférieur), inventor of the guillotine, *Dict. encyclopédique sci. méd.*, 4th ser., 11: 477—79.

7. Genty, "Brillat-Savarin," *Progrès médicale* 34: 386. Jean Gabriel Gallot (1744—94), M. J. Guillaume, ed., *Procès-verbaux du Comité d'instruction publique de l'Assemblée Législative* (Paris, 1889), p.488 (hereinafter cited as *Législative*); *Dict. encyclopédique sci. mèd.*, 4th ser., 6: 542.

8. Jean Baptiste Salle (1759—94) of Vézelize and Pierre Bouisson (1753—1816) of Lauzun. Guillaume, *Convention* 1: xc; 2: xcii; Cabanès, *Evadés*, pp.213—14.

9. *Dict. encyclopédique sci. méd.*, 4th ser., 40: 478; Thompson, *French Revolution*, p.27.

10. George Rudé, *The Crowd in the French Revolution* (Oxford, 1959), pp.34—44.

11. Larrey, *Memoirs* 1:18—19.

12. Norman Hampson, *A Social History of the French Revolution* (London, 1963), p.72; Paul Triaire, *Larrey et les campaigns de la Révolution et de l'Empire, 1768–1842* (Tours, 1902), pp.15–16; McCloy, *Government Assistance*, p.222; *Dict. encyclopédique sci. méd.*, 2d ser., 1: 123.

13. Hampson, *Social History*, p.72; Smeaton, *Fourcroy*, p.39.

14. Soubiran, *Larrey*, p.46; "Dessaix," *Chron. méd.* 16: 700; *Dict. encyclopédique sci. méd.*, 1st ser., 10: 424; 30: 605; 2d ser., 1: 123.

15. Crane Brinton, *The Jacobins: An Essay in the New History* (New York, 1961), p.65.

16. Cabanès, *Costume*, p.33; Paumès, "Parenté médicale," *Chron. méd.* 20: 194; *Dict. encyclopédique sci. méd.*, 3d ser., 12: 705.

17. Laignel-Lavastine, *Histoire générale* 3: 727; Vidal, "Cassanyes," *Révolution française,* 14:968, 996.

18. Cilleuls, "Médecins aux armées," *Revue hist. de l'armée* 6: 15; *Dict. encyclopédique sci. méd.*, 1st ser., 8: 639; 21: 32; 2d ser., 16: 166; Pierre Campmartin (n.d.), Guillaume, *Convention* 1: lxxvii; Christophe Opoix (1745–1840), ibid., 2: xciii; Ferdinand Pierre Marie Dorothée Guille-mardet (1765–1809), ibid., 1: lxxxviii; 2: xciii; Charles Nicolas Beauvais de Préau (1745-93) and Pierre Joseph Duhem (d.1807), ibid., 2: xcii, cii; Léonard Joseph Prunelle de Lière (1748–1828), *Nouvelle biographie* 41: 121. Famous for his violent talk, Duhem said one day when someone cited Jean Jacques Rousseau that he was "an aristocrat and a fanatic, and that he thought that he [Rousseau] would have been a good man to guillotine." Guillaume, *Convention* 3: 488.

19. Louis Alexandre Jard-Panvillier (1757–1822) of Aigonnay, Alphonse Aulard, ed., *Recueil des actes du Comité de salut public* (Paris, 1889–1923), 4: 85; Vidal, "Cassanyes," *Révolution française* 14: 998; René Levasseur (1747–1834) of Sainte Croix and Anne Marie Valdruche (1745–?) of Joinville, Guillaume, *Convention* 2: xcix, ciii; 3: cxxiv; Elie Lacoste (d.1803) of Montignac and Joseph Barthélemy Carrère (1740–?), an emigré, *Nouvelle biographie* 8: 872; 28: 561.

20. Smeaton, *Fourcroy*, pp.38–39; Thompson, *French Revolution*, p.297. Fourcroy was *médecin des pauvres* in the faubourg St. Marceau, one of the poorest quarters of Paris, from 1789 to March 1792.

21. Guillaume, *Législative*, p.488; *Convention* 1: xc; Genty, "Brillat-Savarin," *Progrès médicale* 34: 386; Albert Mathiez, *The French Revolution* (New York, 1929), p.122; *Dict. encyclopédique sci. méd.*, 4th ser., 6: 542.

22. Brinton, *The Jacobins*, p.66; Richard M. Brace, "The Libertarian Crusade of 1792," *Studies in Modern European History in Honor of Franklin Charles Palm* (New York, 1956), p.39; "Dessaix," *Chron. méd.* 16: 700; Ramsay Weston Phipps, *The Armies of the First French Republic and the Rise of the Marshals of Napoleon I* (London,1926–39), 3: 107;

François Amédée Doppet (1753—1810) of Chambéry in Savoy, *Nouvelle biographie* 13: 907—8.

23. Brinton, *The Jacobins*, pp.62—64, 66, 69.

24. Ibid., pp.64, 131; McCloy, *Government Assistance*, p.457.

25. Brinton, *The Jacobins*, p.208.

26. Alphonse Aulard, *Histoire politique de la Révolution* (Paris, 1926), pp.127—29, 153—60.

27. Thompson, *French Revolution*, p.230; Aulard, *Recueil des actes* 4: 85. Pierre Marie Broussonnet (1761—1807) of Montpellier, assistant to Daubenton at the Collége de France, accused as a Girondin, fled to Spain (an emigré), later returned to France under the Directory, *Dict. encyclopédique sci. méd.*, 1st ser., 11: 167. Claude Masuyer, in both the Legislative Assembly and the Convention, arrested and executed in October 1793, Guillaume, *Convention* 1: lxxxvii; René François Plaichard-Choltière (1740—1815), ibid., 2: ci. Jacques René Tenon (1724—1816), *Dict. encyclopédique sci. méd.*, 3d ser., 16: 393.

28. Marie Antoine Baudot (1765—1837) of Charolles, Guillaume, *Convention* 2: xciv—scv; 3: cxxi. Jean Baptiste Bô (1743—1814), a "purifier" of the names of towns; one who hated peasants, had them shot at Aurillac, and told those complaining of food shortages at Cahors, "Relax, twelve million inhabitants will be enough for France, we'll let the rest die." Ibid., 2: xcii. Claude François Siblot (1752—1802), Aulard, *Recueil des actes* 6: 285. Etienne Clédel (1737—1820) of Alvignac, ibid., 18: 403; Jean Guillaume Taillefer (1763—1835) of Domme, ibid., 6: 74—75.

29. Brinton, *Decade of Revolution*, pp.52—59.

30. Ibid., pp.88—90.

31. Jean Pierre Sebastien Mangin (d.1828), Armées du Nord, carton 26, Arch. hist. Service de Santé; Ackernecht, *Paris Hospital*, p.183; "Couthon et Drouet, d'après les 'Souvenirs' d'Isabey," *Chron. méd.* 11: 372; Triaire, *Larrey*, pp.18—19; "Dessaix," *Chron. méd.* 16: 698—700; Guillaume, *Convention* 2: xcii; *Dict. encyclopédique sci. méd.*, 1st ser., 8: 639.

32. Thompson, *French Revolution*, p.312; Guillaume, *Convention* 1: xc, lxxxviii; *Nouvelle biographie* 41: 121; *Dict. encyclopédique sci. méd.* 1st ser., 11: 167.

33. Aulard, *Recueil des actes* 4: 85; Guillaume, *Convention* 1: xc, lxxxvii—lxxxviii; 2: ci; 3: cxxi—cxxii; *Dict. encyclopédique sci. méd.*, 1st ser., 8: 339; 2d ser., 16: 266.

34. Bonnal de Ganges, *Les représentants du peuple en mission près les armées, 1791—1797* (Paris, 1898), 2: 267—69; *Dict. encyclopédique sci. méd.*, 2d ser., 4: 761; 4th ser., 3: 744. Fourcroy took Marat's place in 1793 and sat with the Jacobins. Aulard, *Recueil des actes* 7: 301; Vidal, "Cassanyes," *Révolution française* 14: 968; Guillaume, *Convention* 1: lxxxv; 2: xcii—xciii, xcvii, xcix.

35. Thompson, *French Revolution*, p.297.

36. Georges Pouchet, "Les sciences pendant la Terreur, d'après les documents du temps et les pièces des Archives nationales," *Révolution française* 30: 260.

37. Donald Greer, *The Incidence of the Emigration during the French Revolution* (Cambridge, 1951), pp.86, 134. One of the 587 classified as surgeons and physicians was an oculist.

38. Thompson, *French Revolution*, p.230; *Dict. encyclopédique sci. méd.*, 2d ser., 2: 137; Genty, "Brillat-Savarin," *Progrès médicale* 34: 386.

39. Pierre Poissonier (1720–98) of Dijon and Jacques Philibert Read (1736–96). Cilleuls, " Les médecins aux armées," *Revue hist. de l'armée* 6: 12, 19–21; *Dict. encyclopédique sci. méd.*, 2d ser., 2: 51. Louis Le Monnier (1736–96) of Bouchain (Nord).

40. Laignel-Lavastine, *Histoire générale* 3: 13.

41. Philippe Pinel (1755–1826) of Saint Paul (Tarn), whose most famous work was his *Nosographie philosophique*, 3 vols. (1798). *Nouvelle biographie* 40: 262; *Dict. encyclopédique sci. méd.*, 2d ser., 25: 409; Lester S. King, *The Medical World of the Eighteenth Century* (Chicago, 1958), p.290; Michel Ferron, "Le chirurgien principal de l'armée: Baron Jean Péborde, médecin du Murat," *Progrès médicale* 44: 33; Laignel-Lavastine, *Histoire générale* 2: 340–41; Philippe Jean Pelletan (d.1829), successor to Desault in 1795; Jean Péborde and François Ribes, both future surgeons *par Quartier de l'Empereur* and barons of the Empire; Bernard Bérot, future distinguished professor of physiology at Strasbourg; and Xavier Bichat (1771–1802) of Thiorette, whose *Traité des membranes en générale et des diverses membranes en particulier* (Paris, 1800) launched the science of human tissue.

42. Bichat mentioned his debt to both Corvisart and Desault in his other two works: *Recherches physiologiques sur la vie et la mort* (Paris, 1802), p.345 and *Pathological Anatomy: The Last Course of Xavier Bichat, from an autographic manuscript of P. A. Beclard; with an account of the Life and Labours of Bichat by F. G. Boisseau* (Philadelphia, 1827), p.5; Henri Bon, *Laënnec, 1781–1826* (Dijon, 1925), p.13; Charles J. Singer, *A Short History of Medicine* (New York, 1962), p.172; J. F. H. Dally, "Jean Nicolas Corvisart (1755–1821), Chief Physician to Napoleon I," *Medical Record* 153: 237. René T. H. Laënnec (1781–1826) and Pierre Bretonneau (1771–1862).

43. François Chopart (1743–95) of Paris, named in 1789 as professor of surgery in the School of Surgery, a position he held until his death on June 9, 1795. He apparently died of the same thing that killed Desault (it is still unknown), *Dict. encyclopédique sci. méd.*, 1st ser., 17: 8. Chopart's amputation involved cutting off the forepart of the foot at the metatarsal joint, leaving only the astragalus and calcaneum, and turning under the soft parts of the sole of the foot to form a pad and cover the stump. See

McCloy, *French Inventions*, p.157n.

44. Smeaton, *Fourcroy*, p.20; *Dict. encyclopédique sci. méd.*, 1st ser., 30: 420.

45. Albert Mathiez, "La mobilisation des savants en l'an II," *Revue de Paris* 24: 545; Thompson, *French Revolution*, p.393; Nicolas Dubois de Chémant, *Dissertation sur les avantages des nouvelles dents et rateliers, incorruptibles et sans odeur, inventés* (Paris, 1789), pp.8–9.

46. Larrey, *Memoirs* 1: 25. "These needles were made of fine and highly tempered steel and were of different sizes. The needle was curved into a semi-circle, the extremities being parallel. The point was a small curve with sharp edges, and the edges terminated toward the body in óbtuse angles. The edges were rounded and slightly thinner than the middle of the needle. There was a square, transverse opening through the eye, and a groove, so that a cord or ribbon could lie in it. The advantages that he claimed for these needles were the readiness with which they would pass through the skin and the fact that the ligature would lie free and keep its flattened form, thus supporting the wound edges." J. Chalmers Da Costa, "Baron Larrey," *Johns Hopkins Hosp. Bull.* 17: 199.

47. Laurent, *Percy*, p.60; McCloy, *French Inventions*, pp.162, 166; Thompson, *Surgical Instruments*, p.74.

Chapter Four

DISMANTLING THE OLD REGIME

By January, 1790, the National Assembly was occupied with legislation designed to destroy the institutions of the Old Regime and to create new ones to replace them. As for so many other aspects of French life, revolutionary changes were forecast for medicine. Three separate committees, Health, Education, and Public Welfare, began their studies of how to deal with those three urgent problems, and medicine was implicated in each of them. The Committee on Health was to reorganize medicine's institutions and practices; the Committee on Education was to formulate a new national educational policy, which would also govern medical education. The Committee on Public Welfare, in developing a national approach to the means of relieving the sick, infirm, and aged poor, would certainly require drastic changes in existing French medical institutions and practices.

All three committees were grappling with issues that were of emotional concern to many Frenchmen. The pleas of the *cahiers* and the demands of members of the National Assembly reflected some fundamental convictions: that proper health care, because it related to the poverty and misery of the people, should be available to all through the agency of the State; that education, with a practical curriculum and improved instruction, should be available to all as a doorway to equal opportunity. The decadence and backwardness of education, medicine, and the arts and sciences were viewed as a result of the way the old society had been organized, with its favoritism, misgovernment, maladministration, and general social dislocation. Therefore the privileged academies and corporations, including the Society of Medicine and the Academy of Surgery, were marked for destruction because they symbolized the errors and injustices of the past.

Many of the members of the National Assembly itself were men who were bitterly convinced that their own careers had been limited or stifled by monopolistic and discriminatory practices. Artists such as Louis David and Quatremère de Quincy became self-appointed agents of the destruction of the Royal Academy of Painting and Sculpture.[1] Jean Paul Marat attacked the Royal Academy of Sciences, complaining of its "low persecutions" of him, and in self-revealing phrases declared: "Since the d'Alemberts, the Condorcets, the Moniers, Monges, Lavoisiers and all the other charlatans of that scientific body wanted to hog the limelight for themselves, and since they held the trumpet of fame in their hands, it is not difficult to understand why they disparaged my discoveries throughout Europe, turned every learned society against me, and had all learned publications closed to me . . . . The Revolution announced itself with the convocation of the States-General. I quickly saw how the wind was blowing, and at last I began to breathe in the hope of seeing humanity avenged and myself installed in the place which I deserved . . . ."[2]

Many shared the view of education in France that Lavoisier had expressed: "Public education as it exists in almost the whole of Europe has been devised not with the intention of training citizens but for the purpose of producing priests, monks and theologians."[3] University faculties came under heavy fire because of their privileges, their lingering aura of religion, and their reputed ignorance, especially in medicine. The structure of the old system was antiquated both in its form and goals; it could not satisfy the philosophers' demands for a more practical education and a more virtuous citizenry. The Paris Faculty, for example, had not awarded a doctor's degree since 1785. In 1789 the Royal Society of Medicine admitted that "we must say that in the whole kingdom not a single school exists where the basic principles of the healing art are taught in their totality."[4]

Most of the liberal physicians and surgeons in the National Assembly shared the growing determination to destroy completely the nation's corporate structure. The established Royal Academy of Sciences, the Academy of Surgery, the Society of Medicine, the College of Pharmacy, the Academy of Painting and Sculpture, and all other corporate groups found few defenders, especially among undistinguished, provincial men. Sustained agitation finally brought the issue to a vote in the National Assembly. On August 20, 1790, came the formal demand for the abolition of all academies. Though this resolution was narrowly defeated, government financial support was to be extended to the academies only provisionally, until they rewrote their rules "in consonance with equality," and had them approved by the Assembly.[5]

This action by the National Assembly produced feverish excitement in the academies. The Royal Academy of Surgery quickly renounced its privileges as freely as the nobility had done on the night of August 4–5, 1789. An effort to preserve the tradition whereby the King's first surgeon also served as permanent secretary of the Academy was defeated because it "excluded equality and was repugnant to reason."[6]

A flood of plans for reorganizing medical institutions soon inundated the Assembly. Upon the authorization of the Assembly's Committee of Health, Guillotin had published at public expense his *Projet de décret sur l'enseignement et l'exercise de l'art de guérir* (1790). Other plans for reform of both medical organization and teaching came in from the faculties at Nancy and at Toulouse, and the College of Surgery at Nantes. The Royal Society of Medicine drew up its own plan for the reconstruction of medicine in France, attempting to justify and preserve itself while emphasizing the need to reform the medical schools.[7]

In view of the disarray of military medicine, J. F. Coste prepared and presented a plan for reorganizing the military medical service. As First Physician of the Armies, he had spent most of 1789 making a detailed study of over seventy military hospitals and the effects of the economies put into operation by Jean Colombier's plan. When Coste returned to Paris early in 1790 and was assigned as a consultant to the Committee on Health, his new plan was ready for consideration. Its principal features included a five-member Directory of Health for administration; five medical inspectors-general; equal status as "health officers" for surgeons, pharmacists, and physicians, with all accounting to be done by the health officers (eliminating the war commissioners); and sufficient authority for health officers to police conditions tending to breed bad health or health hazards in any community where the troops were stationed.[8] The sketchy nature of Coste's draft indicates his awareness that the Committee was concerned with a sweeping reform of medicine in general. His report was simply filed away because the Committee intended to concentrate upon Guillotin's broad proposal.

Meanwhile, the Committee on Education held hearings and received proposals for a new educational system for France. Among the outspoken revolutionaries who gave constructive thought to a basic national program of education were Mirabeau, Talleyrand, Condorcet, and Lakanal. Successively, they set out to create a plan that would be equal to the ideals of the Revolution.

It was clear that until the Committee on Education had hammered out an acceptable theory and system of general education, it would offer no specific ideas on the reform of medical teaching and of the medical curriculum. So the established schools of medicine and surgery drifted along, feeling the hostility of their critics and the extreme shortage of money for salaries and other basic operating costs. During 1790 no certificates in surgery were issued, and no examinations given for the degree of *docteur en médecine*.[9] Some private educational institutions reformed themselves. For example, financial difficulties and the emigration of its sponsors led to a reorganization of the Lycée de la Rue Valois where the chemist Fourcroy taught. He now became one of 87 shareholders called "founders" and was elected president on December 21, 1790. His salary, however, was cut from 2,400 to 1,000 livres.[10]

The Committee on Public Welfare, chaired by the Duc de la Rochefoucauld-Liancourt, had undertaken to prepare a complete and thoroughgoing study of all problems relating to poverty and health care, both urban and rural. The Committee was organized into various subcommittees in 1790, and advice and information was solicited and received from a wide variety of sources. Supplementing special reports from the Society of Medicine, the Commissioners undertook a first-hand study by visiting the hospitals and other Paris institutions for the poor to learn what conditions actually were in these places.[11] Liancourt compiled a mass of information and statistics on hospitals and, more generally, on the status of public aid to the poor. The findings of prerevolutionary investigators were confirmed and underscored by all of these reports. Liancourt drafted a program for a complete system of national public assistance and presented it to his committee on December 1, 1790.[12] Once again the role of French medicine, this time in the problem of indigence, had to await clear definition while this plan was discussed and debated.

However, Paris in 1790 was not the place for calm and judicious discussions of how the ideals of the Revolution could best be applied to specific problems. Food riots had begun at Versailles as early as January. Political tension and suspicion were complicated by the soaring cost of living, the fear of famine, and anger at hoarders. Urgent problems demanded solutions, but expedients, rather than real solutions, were sought to handle the crises of the moment. The loud and insistent voices demanding instant reform continued to be heard.

The title *académicien* had become an insult by early 1791. Marat commenced the denunciation of all academies. His *Ami de peuple* of January 27, 1791, contained a vulgar and brutal attack upon Lavoisier. His subsequent pamphlets, including *Les Charlatans modernes*, a diatribe against the Academy of Sciences, denounced Monge, Fourcroy, Laplace, and Beaumé. The Society of Medicine was denounced in the National Assembly for its failure to renounce its privileges as the Academy of Surgery had done. The Assembly soon reacted to these pressures, and on

February 16 abolished the master's degree and all examinations for medical degrees. On March 17, the Assembly decreed that thereafter anyone paying a small fee could be licensed without examination to practice medicine or surgery.[13]

Under the National Assembly's injunction to reform itself, the Royal Society of Medicine finally purged its list of members. At its August 21 meeting, the Society retired Cornette and Carrère to the status of *associés veterans*. From the roster of *associés libres*, the Society decided to remove the names of Amelot, Loménie de Brienne, the Count d'Angivilliers, Breteuil, Lassone, and Le Noir. Of these six, three were emigrés. Loménie de Brienne and Amelot were still in France, but neither had been active in the Society. Lassone was restored at the October 30 meeting where Fourcroy, now a vice-director of the Society, acted as secretary. This same gathering voted to expel the Deans of the Faculty of Medicine of Paris and to purge both Carrère and Cornette because they had emigrated.[14]

Meanwhile, the National Assembly began debate on Guillotin's plan for the reorganization of French medicine. His report, sponsored by the Committee of Health, was accepted after much discussion. As passed by the Assembly, including amendments, the new law proposed that medical instruction be reestablished at Paris, Strasbourg, Bordeaux, and Montpellier. In addition, it called for the creation of an agency of health in each of the new districts (*arondissements*), charged with responsibility for hygiene and public health. This legislation, however, was faulty because these agencies were given neither authority nor funds; predictably, nothing happened.[15]

The makers of the new Constitution of September 3, 1791, contented themselves with the hope that "there will be created and organized a general establishment to provide for orphans and foundlings, to care for the sick and infirm poor, and to provide work for the indigent."[16] Vainly Liancourt attempted to get the National Assembly to discuss his plan for health care and public assistance. Pointing to the desperate financial plight of the hospitals since the abolition of the *octroi*, he continued to plead for constructive action through the closing days of the Assembly. However, when adjournment *sine die* came on September 30, the political careers of Liancourt and Guillotin were over, and the incoming Legislative Assembly inherited the unsolved problems of health care, education, and public welfare.[17]

The National Assembly's failure to enact positive legislation was especially disastrous for French hospitals. The economic depression, which had been deepening since 1787, initiated a decline in hospital revenues.

The political upheaval of 1789, which abolished feudal dues, rents, and fees, especially the *dîme*, further weakened chronically precarious hospital finances. Another blow of staggering proportions was the decree of November 2, 1789. By seizing all church properties for national use, the Assembly eased the government's financial crisis but paralyzed many hospitals operated by religious groups and others deriving their chief income from church lands. The demoralization of hospital personnel grew after the Assembly suppressed monastic vows on February 13, 1790, and ordered an end to cloistered life from some 300,000 monks and nuns. Although this did not produce the violent resistance that followed later laws affecting the secular clergy, many small hospitals attached to religious cloisters became scenes of bitter quarrels between local authorities and the former monks and nuns.[18]

Some hospital personnel experienced great difficulty in adjusting to the equality of being "health officers," a term borrowed from the military service and applied by the revolutionaries to physicians, surgeons, apothecaries, and hospital administrators alike. Hospitals became *hospices*, and the urge to eradicate all vestiges of the Old Regime usually led local authorities to rename the Hôtel-Dieu the "*Hospice d'humanité*" and the Charité the "*Hospice de bienfaisance*."

In the unstable political climate, three factors were operating to make the financial distress of hospitals even more acute: the smaller return on the monetary investments they held, the diminishing support of private philanthropists, and the inability or unwillingness of many Frenchmen to pay their taxes.[19] After January 1, 1791, all hospitals were required to pay a tax on all their landed property. The result was a reduction of normal hospital revenues by at least 20 percent. In March, the National Assembly's abolition of direct taxes again bit into hospital income, and the suppression of the *octroi* on May 1 completed the wreckage of hospital finances. In their haste to end many old tax inequities, the revolutionary legislators had overlooked the fact that the chief revenue tax for hospital poor relief was the *octroi* on wine.[20]

The Assembly belatedly sought to discover exactly what had happened to hospitals as a result of its legislation. It charged the committees of Health and Public Welfare to make a study during the spring of 1791. These committees found that the revenue of the Paris hospitals had dropped from 7,958,799 livres in 1788 to 4,129,206 livres in 1790, and that the income of over 1,400 hospitals had fallen from 20,874,665 livres to 13,987,788 livres.[21] These statistics prompted the Assembly on April 10 to appropriate 76,396 livres as compensation for several hospitals that had lost revenue due to the new tax but an immediate flood of similar claims established the total inadequacy of this fund.[22] Ten days later, the Assembly took another approach and stopped the sale of church lands that were producing income for hospitals. However, property already sold and revenues lost in consequence were irretrievable.[23]

Meanwhile, the committees collected 1,438 completed questionnaires from a total of 2,185 hospitals. Although some conditions were uncovered that were even more horrifying than those reported by Tenon in 1788, the committees were content to make only some recommendations about better ventilation in the wards and individual beds for the patients. Regarding the problem of finances, except for a few scattered calls for government confiscation of hospitals, no recommendations were formulated to try to ease the deep financial crisis of the hospitals.[24]

The National Assembly, occupied with trying to launch the Constitution of 1791 and hampered by a reluctant Louis XVI, resorted simply to the expedient of more hospital subsidies. Inundated by pleas and protests, it established a loan fund of three million livres on July 25, but this fund was exhausted by September 12. Slated to die on September 30, the Assembly simply turned out another grant of one and one-half million livres.[25]

With the convening of the new Legislative Assembly in October, the problems of the Revolution mounted. Hospital troubles in the autumn of 1791 were compounded by efforts to enforce the Civil Constitution of the Clergy, wide resistance to the requirement that secular clergy take an oath of allegiance, and an increasingly militant anti-clericalism. Typical of the new, zealous municipal authorities were those at Valognes (Manche) who tried to force the nonjuring priests and nuns from the hospital by closing its chapel. Bitter, paralyzing quarrels in local hospitals spread over the country, involving administrators, physicians, surgeons, and various religious and lay groups that provided the essential nursing service. At Port Louis (Morbihan), hospital authorities who attempted to require all the staff to take the civil oath faced a mass walk-out by the Sisters of Wisdom. Patients there went completely without care until the administrators temporarily abandoned the oath, reopened the chapel, and reinstated the nonjuring priest of the hospital. Elsewhere, the Sisters of Charity, the largest group serving hospitals, refused to disband. They petitioned for funds, and continued to operate their hospices for orphans and for the sick.[26]

While the new committees of Public Education, Health, and Welfare picked up studies made by their predecessors in the National Assembly, the Legislative Assembly bought time in the hospital crisis. On January 22, 1792, it voted another one and one-half million livres as an emergency loan to hospitals. Two weeks later, trying to move toward a more permanent solution to the rapidly developing chaos in health care the Legislative Assembly decreed that rents due hospitals had been "forgiven" only for 1791 and would have to be paid in 1792. It was hoped that the religious quarrels would be settled by a decree of April 6 which abolished "all religious corporations and secular congregations of men and women, ecclesiastical or lay, even those uniquely devoted to the service of hospitals and to the comfort of the sick . . .".[27]

The Legislative Assembly was distinctly more hostile to old corporations and academies than the National Assembly had been. Reluctantly, representatives of the medical profession approached the Legislative Assembly requesting that it do something about the shocking conditions in medical degrees. With the profession wide open to anyone able to buy a license, on January 8, 1792, "several members of the College of Surgery asked for an explanation, regarding their profession, of the Law of March 17 [1791] which abolished the master's degree and the examining juries, by establishing a license."[28] The Legislative Assembly simply referred this meek petition to its Committee of Public Education and nothing further was done.

With war imminent, a stronger effort was made on April 2 to end this indiscriminate licensing in the medical profession. Jean Maugras, representing the College of Surgery, appeared before the Committee of Public Education. He first inquired as to whether already established surgeons would have to pay for licences and then discreetly asked the Committee "if it would not be inconvenient to issue licenses indiscriminately, without the candidates submitting some proof to assure the degree of their instruction."[29] Whatever good effect this mild approach might have had was ruined by two petitions presented later at the same hearing. Paris physicians asked exemption from the new Law of Patents because they did not want to reveal the ingredients of their secret remedies. Then the old corporation of master apothecaries, the College of Pharmacy, undiplomatically presented a protest against "the extreme and dangerous ease with which the City distributed licenses of the professions."[30]

Reaction was swift and sharp in the Committee. The physicians and surgeons were told bluntly that all the professions were "equal in talents and virtues" and that all of them would have to submit to the patent regulations and pay the tax just like anyone else. One member of the Committee urged that the petition of the College of Pharmacy be combined with that made by Maugras for the College of Surgery, "being similar in their object, which is to maintain both of these [institutions] as shelters for the abuses of ignorance and the audacity of charlatanism."[31]

The motion carried and the combined petition was referred to a joint committee of Finance, Liquidation, and Public Health, and thus buried.

On April 20, 1792, the long-awaited report on the new organization of public education was presented to the Legislative Assembly by Condorcet. The section on medical instruction offered no comfort to the academies. Condorcet had placed medicine and surgery in a classification called "The Application of Sciences to the Arts," including agriculture, construction arts, hydraulics, navigation, machines and instruments, mechanical arts, and chemical arts. All academies, faculties, and universities were to be absorbed into the architechtonic national educational system that Condorcet proposed. He was briefly interrupted on April 20 so that the Legislative Assembly could declare war on Austria, but after this distraction Condorcet proceeded to summarize his vision of the new system of medical education: "While the elementary theory of the medical sciences will be taught in the departmental institutes, the hospital doctors will teach, practice, and give lessons in surgery; in this way the schools where one will receive elementary knowledge will be multiplied and will assure the poor of the aid of enlightened men, developed by a good method, instructed in the art of observation, and free from the prejudices and ignorance of those in the systematic doctrines."[32]

With war under way, the oldest and most respected of all academies, the Academy of Sciences, came under heavy attack. On April 25, the militant Fourcroy rose in the academy's meeting and proposed that it follow the example of the Society of Medicine and purge its membership of all who were "counter-revolutionaries" and all who had left the country. Fourcroy's resolution was defeated, but the Academy of Sciences took every other possible means to avoid an appearance of lack of sympathy with the Revolution. It voted a "patriotic gift" to the nation of 11,845 livres, plus a piece of gold valued at 12,000 livres.[33]

Nevertheless, the inexorable movement of the foes of all corporate institutions left over from the Old Regime continued. By August 18, 1792, complete suppression of the universities and all faculties of medicine had been decreed by the Legislative Assembly. Hoping to avoid a similar fate, the members of the Academy of Sciences frantically pulled down the tapestries in their meeting place in the Louvre, explaining that they did not want to display "symbols that should be banished from a republican country."[34]

Distinguished individuals like Desault, who was far more concerned with surgery than politics, were harassed. Desault's students at the Hôtel-Dieu sought to ease the pressure on their teacher by appearing before the Legislative Assembly on August 28, "paying homage to his virtue in order to protest all the calumnies spread against him." They took the oath of allegiance and offered to "give their services to their brave brothers-in-arms in the army encamped at Paris and who go to fight for liberty."[35] The next week, during the bloody September Massacres, they reappeared before the Legislative Assembly, offering to form a volunteer company to serve their country, either as soldiers or as surgeons. At the same time, they deposited "on the altar of the country" 2,644 livres and 2 sous for the war effort, carefully stressing that it was a collection "to which M. Desaux [sic] surgeon-major of the Hôtel-Dieu had contributed the sum of 600 livres."[36]

The Legislative Assembly's Committee of Public Education was still struggling to produce a workable system of education. It is indicative of the confusion toward the close of the Legislative Assembly that there was a debate as to whether medical instruction in the colleges should not exist simply to allow citizens to satisfy their curiosity. The Committee wondered if this sort of instruction "could be considered sufficient proof for those who wanted to practice medicine." The discussion produced only the obvious conclusion that aspiring practitioners "will have to have more instruction in practical medicine; the means by which it will be done is to be determined by the Committee of Public Education in joint session with that of Welfare."[37] The work of reorganizing medical instruction was still unfinished when the Legislative Assembly dissolved and the new National Convention assembled on September 22, 1792.

As the Convention's Committee of Public Education began its work on the problem, Navier and Quatremère de Quincy were vigorously demanding the suppression of all French academies. David joined them on November 11, when he delivered a biting condemnation of the Academy of Painting and Sculpture and heaped odium upon all academicians. By November 25, David was supported by G. Romme, the two presenting a call for "no half-measures," demanding "that the same blow should strike all the academies in France."[38] Although he was a member of the Committee of Public Education, which had approved Condorcet's plan, Romme opposed it before the Convention on December 20. He delivered a wild attack upon all academicians for their petty jealousies, eternal feuds, and public quarrels. "Nominations," Romme declared, "have nearly always been an element of intrigue and a subject of scandal, in giving prizes to baseness and audacity rather than merit, and to favor rather than justice."[39]

Advocating a system of medical instruction involving a five-year program in departmental institutes alone, Romme argued that "good country doctors" would thus be produced. He told those who were hoping to preserve the Society of Medicine: "Medicine, great and sublime in its object, imposing by its numerous relations which attach it to nearly all branches of human knowledge, but often unfortunate in its practice, is vain, fastidious, and nearly null in its teaching; it is unbalanced in its emphases, too glib with the powers it controls, unjustly inequitable and often venal in its works, mysteriously unrighteous in its hieroglyphic formulas and barbaric in their language even though they are French."[40]

Durand Maillaine, another member of the Committee of Public Education, widened the issue into an attack upon all teachers, representing them as "a formidable corporation in the republic." He protested: "It is very strange that, under the pretext of science and enlightenment, they [the Committee of Public Education] propose to the nation to make, at its own expense, a particular and permanent estate of a class of citizens; and what citizens? Men the most capable of swaying public opinion in their direction, because there is a superstition for those called savants, just as there is one for kings and for priests; I refer to those in our most celebrated academies . . . ."[41]

The increasingly violent tempo and broader scope of the Jacobin attack so demoralized the Society of Medicine that it virtually ceased to function after 1792. To this point in the Revolution only a few individuals in the medical profession had been subjected to any personal abuse. The principal focus of the assault was still upon privileged corporations, academies, and monopolies held over from the Old Regime. The abolition of all of these institutions now seemed to be inevitable.

The declaration of war on April 20, 1792, had forced the Legislative Assembly to act to preserve hospital facilities for military use. It ordered the Committee of Health and Public Welfare to study and report on a new hospital organization for the nation and, in the interim, decreed on May 2 that "in the hospitals and houses of charity, the same persons will continue as before the service and comfort of the sick, as individuals, under surveillance of municipal and administrative bodies."[42] However, this attempt to "freeze" the religious and lay orders in the hospital service was but a temporary war measure. The attack upon the congregations was followed by a systematic effort to replace their members as individuals. Despite the chaotic conditions in the hospitals and the urgent need to establish an orderly system, the Legislative Assembly took steps on September 19 to replace experienced nursing personnel. It ordered that "the widows and orphans of the defenders of the nation, killed in war, will be given preference in employment for service in the infirmaries and military hospitals."[43]

Three days later, this policy was confirmed when the new National

Convention convened in Paris. The Convention also pursued the course previously set toward national organization, administration, and regulation of all hospitals in France. War had now diverted funds from charities, and the Convention further diminished hospital revenues by abolishing lotteries on November 30, 1792. At the same time, provision was made for state subsidization: "Hospitals and houses of charity which, by the suppression of lotteries, shall have lost part or all of their support, will receive provisional help from the Minister of the Interior, upon request of the administrative bodies, which will declare the actual loss and needs of the said houses."[44] In a steady movement toward centralization of the hospital system, the Convention voted two subsidies to hospitals, the first, of 8 million livres, on July 14, 1793, a second of 10 million livres on February 1, 1794. The logical conclusion of steps taken since 1789 was the decree of July 11, 1794, which transferred all hospital properties to the state and announced the nation's assumption of responsibility for all hospital expenses.[45]

In recasting the old hospital system, revolutionary policies of steadily cutting into hospital revenues and of ousting members of religious groups from the hospitals were offset by policies of subsidy and of employment in hospitals on the basis of patriotism. In both cases, the results were unfortunate. As widows and orphans of deceased veterans replaced experienced nursing personnel, the quality of hospital service declined sharply. Although initial subsidies of four and one-half million livres made in 1791 and again in 1792 were increased to eight million in 1793 and to ten million in 1794, the increases were more than offset by inflation, and hospital finances continued to be inadequate. The nation was still faced with the task of trying to make up the difference between the thirty million livre income that hospitals had enjoyed before 1789 and the estimated three to four million to which that income had shrunk. The net effect of revolutionary legislation in this period was disastrous. It permitted hospitals to sink into a state of decay and neglect far worse than that which had existed before the Revolution.

The army medical service had not fared well during this period, either. The 1788 legislation, which had reduced the large teaching hospitals to "auxiliary" status while pushing the creation of regimental hospitals, failed of implementation during the first two years of the Revolution, despite the indefatigable work of J. F. Coste and Pierre Percy. With pay in arrears as much as eighteen months, many physicians and surgeons returned to civilian practice. The number of "health officers" in the service fell from 1,200 in 1788 to the neighborhood of 200 during 1789–90. The medical service continued to be torn by the three-cornered rivalry of the physicians, surgeons, and war commissioners.[46] Consequently, the facilities and the personnel available to serve the armies of the Republic in 1791 were not sufficient for peacetime needs, much less for wartime demands.

The planned increase in military forces in 1791 was 169 battalions of volunteers (101,000 men). Only 60 battalions were organized by September 25 and even by January, 1792, France was still 51,000 men short of this goal. Yet even these numbers placed a heavy strain upon the inadequate existing military medical service. In an effort to provide the armies with the needed medical personnel, on September 20, 1791, the National Assembly required military commanders to cooperate directly with the medical chiefs of each army in the procurement of physicians, surgeons, apothecaries, and nursing staffs. The same decree severely limited the authority of the old war commissioners, whose loyalty was now suspect.[47]

The task of recruiting medical personnel of quality was not eased by the law of October 16 which required a surgeon-major for each company of National Guards bound for frontier defense. This requirement was nullified by the ease with which charlatans and amateurs could purchase licenses to practice medicine and surgery. The Legislative Assembly in late 1791 had to give the chief health officers of the armies the direction of all military hospitals, as well as complete supervision of their personnel. Some effort was made to screen employees and military medical officers and their assistants, but poorly trained and incapable men continued to enter the medical service during 1791—a factor that led to a return to procedures used before the Revolution. As war approached in early 1792, the army's Council of Health was reestablished by the Legislative Assembly and given wide powers. Its function was to screen and recommend medical men to the Minister of War who issued their commissions, provided the applicants held the proper certificates of patriotism.[48]

One of the applicants who won a commission was C. A. Lombard, Jr., son of the former surgeon-in-chief of civilian and military hospitals. He was a volunteer assigned to the mobile hospitals of the Army of the Rhine on August 7, 1791. During the winter of 1791—92, the 18-year-old Lombard completed a course in surgery at Strasbourg. His eight-page, handwritten examination (dated April 1, 1792) reveals much both about the young surgeon and about the Republic's need for military surgeons. The first question asked for comments upon the methods being used to insure the competence of health officers, to which Lombard wrote in reply a two-page essay declaring that too many imcompetents were being commissioned! The second question was a very elementary one on wound-bandaging. But the third question dealt with aneurism (the ballooning of an artery, usually fatal unless corrected by the most highly skilled surgical specialist): "They diagnose aneurism; they decide that an operation for this illness is necessary, so what procedure do you advise? " Lombard's reply began, "The answer is most elementary," and he proceeded to outline surgical measures certain to be fatal! Having passed the examination, Lombard was assigned to the Army of the Rhine as a surgeon first-class.[49]

By the time war was declared on April 20, some 1,400 physicians and surgeons had volunteered to serve. The Legislative Assembly did not even enact legislation that authorized the establishment of fixed hospitals and the creation of army field hospitals until April 27. In this emergency, the initiative and authority of chief health officers were augmented. The effective functioning of the military medical service was to be assured by having chief health officers directly responsible to army commanders, who were authorized to requisition and confiscate whatever the medical officers required. The Legislative Assembly authorized the requisitioning of public and private buildings, chateaux, émigré homes, convents, and churches, together with any of the material or movable property they contained. By the Law of April 27, 1792, the Provisional Executive Council was instructed by the Legislative Assembly to proceed to "draft a regulation which will contain all details of the health service, as well as the administration and cleanliness of the said hospitals: it will fix the service ranks, the functions of the different health officers, their employees and servants, their discipline and their reports; it will determine the rules to be established and the regimen of the patients and the prescriptions of the health officers, the method of supervision; and, finally, the forms to be followed for the general and particular accountability and administration of these establishments."[50]

This Law of April 27 revealed much about the Republic's shocking lack of preparation for war. The Legislative Assembly had merely sketched the barest outlines of a military medical service that would have to be created under revolutionary and wartime conditions. The hospitals, both civil and military, were in the most chaotic condition. By the spring of 1792, the few that were operating did so with demoralized administrations, inexperienced nursing staffs, and almost nonexistent revenues. The continuing attack upon lay and religious hospital corporations, university medical faculties, and the academies had an extremely disquieting effect upon the medical service. Its personnel, swollen by the volunteers of 1791, included unfrocked monks, amateur physicians, and students.[51] The

Legislative Assembly did not even set up a table of rank or a scale of pay and authorized no funds for permanent military hospitals until September 3, 1792.[52] Although medical men enjoyed their new freedom from the war commissioners, and responded well when war was declared in the spring of 1792, the Legislative Assembly offered them practically nothing. There were no funds, no available supplies, no established regimental or field hospitals, and incompetent physicians and surgeons were mobilized along with the competent. The requisitioning of men and supplies produced unending confusion. Throughout most of 1792, the nature of French medicine in the armies of the Republic was that of a grand and desperate improvisation, the handiwork of veteran army officers and top military medical men in the field.

NOTES

1. David L. Dowd, "Art and Politics during the French Revolution: A Study of Three Artist Regicides," *Studies in Modern European History in Honor of Franklin Charles Palm*, p.110.

2. Quoted in Stanley Loomis, *Paris in the Terror, June 1793–July 1794* (Philadelphia, 1964), p.85. The "discoveries" referred to are to be found in *Découvertes de M. Marat sur la Lumière* (Paris, 1780), *Recherches physiques sur la feu* (Paris, 1780), and *Recherches physiques sur l'électricité; par M. Marat, Docteur en Médecine des Gardes du Corps de Monseigneur le Comte d'Artois* (Paris, 1782).

3. Denis Duveen, "Antoine Laurent Lavoisier and the French Revolution," *Journal of Chemical Education* 31: 61.

4. Quoted in Ackernecht, *Paris Hospital*, p.31.

5. *Arch. parl.* 42: 175; Fayet, *La Révolution et la science*, p.121.

6. Laignel-Lavastine, *Histoire générale* 2: 447.

7. Guillaume, *Législative*, p.viii; *Convention* 2: 86.

8. Coste dossier, carton 205/1, Val-de-Grâce.

9. Cabanès, *Chirurgiens et blessés*, p.310.

10. Smeaton, *Fourcroy*, p.16.

11. Rosen, "Hospitals, Medical Care and Social Policy," *Bull. Hist. Med.* 30: 131.

12. Camille Bloch and Alexandre Tuetey, eds., *Procès-verbaux et rapports du Comité de Mendicité de la Constituante, 1790–1797* (Paris, 1911), pp.575–693 (hereinafter cited as *Comité de Mendicité*).

13. Guillaume, *Convention* 2: 85; Laignel-Lavastine, *Histoire générale* 3: 727.

14. Smeaton, *Fourcroy*, pp.23, 45–46; *Nouvelle biographie* 8: 872–73.

15. Laignel-Lavastine, *Histoire générale* 3: 496–97.

16. J. M. Thompson, ed., *French Revolution Documents, 1789–1794* (London, 1933), p.113.

17. Rosen, "Hospitals, Medical Care and Social Policy," *Bull. Hist. Med.* 30: 137.

18. Joseph Clémanceau, "Notes sur les Etats-Généraux et l'Assemblée constituante," *Revue historique de la Révolution française* 12: 129.

19. Guillaume, *Législative*, pp.x–xi; McCloy, *Government Assistance*, pp.199, 237.

20. *Arch. parl.* 56: 607, 618, 642.

21. McCloy, *Government Assistance*, p.208.

22. *Arch. parl.* 49: 17–20.

23. Clémanceau, "Notes," *Revue hist. Rév. française* 12: 129.

24. McCloy, *Government Assistance*, p.208.

25. *Arch. parl.* 49: 17–20; 56: 642–43.

26. Guillaume, *Législative*, pp.385–87, 393, 399–401.

27. Ibid, pp.170–71; *Arch. parl.* 38: 273; 56: 643.

28. *Arch. parl.* 25: 61; Guillaume, *Législative*, p.132.

29. Jean Baptiste Maugras (1762–1830) of Fresnes, *Nouvelle biographie* 34: 353; Guillaume, *Législative*, p.165.

30. *Arch. parl.* 41: 762; 42: 41–42.

31. Guillaume, *Convention* 2: 86n.1.

32. Guillaume, *Législative*, p.204.

33. Mathiez, "Mobilisation des savants," *Revue de Paris* 24: 547; McKie, *Lavoisier*, pp.358, 362.

34. Laignel-Lavastine, *Histoire générale* 3: 468.

35. *Arch. parl.* 49: 73.

36. Ibid., 49: 241.

37. Guillaume, *Législative*, p.180.

38. *Arch. parl.* 53: 364, 578–79.

39. Guillaume, *Convention* 1: 204.

40. Ibid., 1: 202, 211–12.

41. Ibid., 1: 123.

42. Guillaume, *Législative*, p.275.

43. *Arch. parl.* 50: 146.

44. Guillaume, *Convention* 1: 104.

45. *Arch. parl.* 56: 644.

46. Laurent, *Percy*, p.5; Triaire, *Larrey*, pp.50–51; Cabanès, *Chirurgiens et blessés*, pp.334, 336.

47. Samuel F. Scott, "The Regeneration of the Line Army during the French Revolution," *Journal of Modern History* 42: 324–26; Phipps,

Armies of the First Republic 1: 15—16; Albert Mathiez, "La mobilisation générale en l'an II, " *Revue de Paris* 24: 584—85.

48. Laws and Decrees, carton 1, Arch. hist. Service de Santé; Cabanès, *Chirurgiens et blessés*, pp.338, 344.

49. Lombard dossier, carton 209/1, Val-de-Grâce. Lombard was later commended for valor by Chief Quartermaster Villemanzy and promoted to surgeon-aide-major in August, 1793.

50. *Arch. parl.* 42: 455—56.

51. *Réimpression de l'ancien Moniteur* [*universel*], *seule histoire authentique et inaltérée de la Révolution française depuis la réunion des Etats-Généraux jusqu'au Consulat (mai 1789—novembre 1799), avec des notes explicatives* 32 vols. (Paris, 1847—50), 9: 791 (hereinafter cited as *Moniteur*). For the first time given the rights of active citizens on September 27, 1791, Jews entered the medical profession along with hundreds of other untrained Frenchmen who paid the fee for a license.

52. *Arch. parl.* 49: 329—30; Bottet, "Le passé," *Caducée* 5: 151.

Chapter Five

IMPROVISING A MILITARY
MEDICAL SERVICE, 1792-1793

Early in 1792, when the French armies began to put together a medical service in anticipation of a declaration of war, the top positions went to experienced physicians and surgeons who had served with distinction in the armies of the Old Regime. These veteran French medical men were asked to assume repsonsibility for training military physicians and surgeons, the staffing of military hospitals, and the procurement of medicines, bandages, bedding, and transport.

One by one they donned their old uniforms once again. In January, J. F. Coste resigned as mayor of Versailles, pulled on white stockings, white linen trousers (now a little tight), and put on a gray cloth vest and frock-coat. The black velvet lapels of his coat displayed two embroidered gold stars, and the cuffs and pocket flaps were trimmed with a double row of gold braid, signifying Coste's position as chief medical inspector of the Armies. André Dufresnoy, at Metz, was also entitled to two gold stars as physician-in-chief of the Army of the North but merited only a single line of gold braid. New uniforms, identical to Dufresnoy's, were worn by J. A. Lorentz (Army of the Rhine) and P. C. Gorcy, physician-in-chief of the Army of the Sambre-et-Meuse.[1]

In token of the continuing supremacy of the physicians, surgeons were not entitled to gold stars. As consulting surgeon of the armies of the North and of the Moselle, Sabatier wore just two rows of gold braid on his coat and three gold buttons on each pocket flap. The crimson velvet lapels on his gray frock-coat and his scarlet vest marked him as a surgeon. C. A. Lombard, with the armies of the Rhine and Sambre-et-Meuse, was dressed identically. The surgeons-in-chief of these armies merited no gold braid at all. The uniforms of C. B. LaGresie (North), J. F. Thomassin (Rhine), and Nicolas Saucerotte (Sambre-et-Meuse) had gold buttons, scarlet vests, and crimson coat lapels, but P. F. Percy, with perverse delight, wore a plain gray uniform as surgeon-in-chief of the Army of the Moselle. A. M.

Parmentier, pharmacist-in-chief of the Armies, wore a scarlet vest and a gray frock-coat with green lapels which identified the military pharmacists. The uniforms of all of these medical officers were rounded out by three-cornered hats, dragoon's swords, and boots.[2]

Despite the fact that the military hospitals had been abolished and their personnel dispersed, there were still some good military physicians and surgeons in the few regimental hospitals. The declaration of war on April 20, 1792, made the recruiting of other good health officers possible, even though the medical service was badly disorganized. In the lower ranks, however, many were brought in who had had only short periods of medical study and possessed only the vaguest notions of military medicine. Among them were former students of theology and law, as well as monks who had been thrown out of cloistered life by a revolutionary decree. The critical condition of the military medical service called for improvisation in almost everything. The veteran medical officers therefore tried to use the spring and summer of 1792 to piece together a viable medical service for each army, to equip each health officer, and to instruct all novices in the art of military medicine.

The distinguished veteran Coste seemed to have the confidence of everyone. He had been widely praised by George Washington for his services in America and was the recipient of an honorary degree from the University of Pennsylvania in 1782. Coste had even been lauded by Voltaire, who referred to him as "notre médecin trés-amiable" in a letter to the Duc de Choiseul.[3] His hospital study of 1789, his service as consultant to the National Assembly's Committee on Health, and his popularity as mayor of Versailles had made Coste the logical choice to head the military medical service in 1792. Once war was declared, the Committee on Health looked to Coste for a detailed inspection of the actual state of the medical service. He was given tremendous responsibility and wide authority in July of 1792 to "interview physicians, surgeons, hospital administrators; judge their general effectiveness; observe the capacity to move sick and wounded; inspect the hospital pharmacies, bakeries, and the quality of food and wine; insure fresh air and whitewashed walls; set up teaching facilities in the large hospitals and explain the proper conduct of health officers; and provide special facilities for venereals."[4]

Selected to act with Coste in this extraordinary assignment were Parmentier and Sabatier. It took them just four months, to the end of November, 1792, to complete their inspection of the armies and hospitals from Calais to Strasbourg. The reports furnished to the Committee of Health during this period were meticulously detailed. In addition to written summaries, the three inspectors devised printed report forms. For example, one form of ten columns provided information on physicians, surgeons, and other hospital personnel as follows: position held, name, age, birth information, previous service, length of service in present position, name of the person who secured or assigned them their places, notes—divided into two subcolumns headed "Talents" and "Patriotism," performance rating, and other observations.[5] Another set of forms provided a comprehensive inventory of drugs, itemizing everything on hand and indicating what was "urgently needed."[6]

A third standard form reported on the patients, with lines to indicate the numbers in the hospital on the first of the month, entering during the month, dismissed, and died. These figures were broken down into four columns headed *fever, wounded, itch* and *venereals.* For example, at Dunkerque on November 26, 1792, 99 soldiers had fevers, 67 were wounded, 20 had the itch, and 81 were venereals. The illnesses of 36 were undiagnosed and 3 had died, all with fever. At Berquere, two days later, there were 57 with fever, 31 wounded, 26 with the itch, and 11 venereals, with 5 dead of fever and 14 undiagnosed.[7] These three forms became the regulation report forms in the armies and hospitals after 1792.

Although they could not know how brief it would be, to energetic and talented military medical men like Coste, Sabatier, and Parmentier, the year 1792 was the beginning of a golden age. They had been freed from the control of the war commissioners by the Council of Health's decree of February 28, which authorized their "working directly with army commanders in setting up the military medical service."[8] The decree of April 18 gave regular army officer rank to medical men, a free hand in medical decision-making, and the decisive voice in planning and executing medical care for the sick and wounded of the armies. A June decree, designed to end graft and profiteering by contractors, authorized free treatment in military hospitals and promised government-furnished provisions and medical supplies.[9] This promise went unfulfilled, but the aggressive medical officers did not hesitate to use the army's power to requisition and confiscate whatever they needed during the critical last six months of 1792.

Wherever it was necessary to establish new hospital facilities, the careful records kept by Coste, Sabatier, and Parmentier enabled them to requisition supplies from hospitals with surpluses and to order the essential medical men from other places to staff them. Incompetent hospital administrators were summarily dismissed, compulsory instruction was established to train the inexperienced medical assistants, standardized hospital regulations were laid down, and Coste's steely gaze made it clear to all hospital personnel that negligence, inefficiency, or malpractice would meet with dismissal and military discipline. Where there were no military hospitals, civilian facilities were requisitioned. By the end of 1792, these three chief medical inspectors had, along a great arc defended by the armies of the North, the Center, and the Rhine, "produced the first really standardized organization of medical services in the hospitals of these armies."[10]

The organization of medical services for each army had been under way simultaneously. P. F. Percy, who had replaced Sabatier as Consulting Surgeon of the Army of the North, reported to Valenciennes in June, 1792. He immediately set about the task of equipping his battle surgeons. Each was given his own personal equipment. A black morocco box was standard issue. Divided into compartments, it contained a case of surgical instruments, some medicines, and other articles designed for use in the field. Bandages, tourniquets, and sutures were included as well as various suture needles of poor design and, often, of defective steel. A simple probe, a pair of surgical tweezers, a pair of surgical scissors, and a pair of large dressing forceps were in each instrument case. There was also a scalpel with a leaf-shaped blade riveted to a shaped bone handle and a crescent-shaped amputation knife. To carry in his coat pocket, each man was issued a small leather bottle of sweet spirits of wine.[11]

Physicians, on the other hand, brought their own bags of pills and potions. When their personal supplies ran out, they expected to find replacements in the hospital pharmacies. Percy, who could not conceal his contempt for physicians, influenced some of his subordinates to drop all unnecessary contraptions and complicated medicines, but the military physicians were afraid of losing their reputations if they ceased to prescribe their secret preparations. When typhus broke out in the camps of the Army of the Moselle in the late summer of 1792, Percy promptly attributed its deadly effects to the medicines administered by the physicians. Terming the prescriptions "murderers," Percy took over all typhus victims at Trarbach on the Moselle in August, 1792, put them in isolation in empty houses, fed them well, and smugly watched them recover.[12]

The war had been delayed, except for a few skirmishes, while Prussia joined Russia in the second partition of Poland. While the French armies waited they tried to combine into an effective fighting force the volunteers of 1791, the levies of 1792, and troops of the line who still retained their aristocratic white uniforms. The absence of any orderly recruiting system resulted in widespread indiscipline. Officers complained of being sent "thieves and malingerers." The 12th Battalion of the Haute-Saône was reportedly made up of boys from thirteen to fourteen years of age.[13] The 3rd Paris Battalion with the Army of the North was described by its commander as unfit for service: "Some of them are attacked by incurable diseases, others are imbeciles, others are blind, infirm, or drunkards. Some are too old, others are too young and too weak ... others are, finally, so small that their guns top their heads by a full foot."[14] The levies of 1792 had evidently induced the towns and villages to send the armies many of their misfits and health problems.

Even before the heavy fighting began, the military hospitals were filling up with unfit troops. Inactivity during the summer allowed the development of the traditional army of women camp-followers, so that Briot was soon able to say confidently that he "had no reason to doubt that at least one-fourth of the soldiers were subject to gonorrhea and syphilis."[15] In addition to the soldiers who had contracted typhus and venereal disease, by August there were growing numbers of men suffering from fevers and dysentery. Lafont-Gouzi noted that most of the dysentery cases seen by the health officers were usually far advanced. He complained that "as the fever associated with diarrhea dominated the second week, it was often very difficult to know which of the two you had to combat."[16] Two other major afflictions were lice and the itch. The latter was endemic in Lorraine and Franche-Comté, and it spread rapidly through the armies encamped near there. Briot estimated in 1792 that one-tenth of the effective troops would be lost due to the itch alone.[17] Lice were a constant problem. One encamped volunteer of 1792 wrote home to his parents: "We have two beds for five men; it was decided by lot that I would be in the bed with three persons. Our bed is made of straw, with a sheet thrown over it. Over the sheet, a down comfort of covering. That would not be so bad but for the fact that all the detachments are bedded time after time on the same sheets. *There are also lice* but let's not talk of that."[18]

With the Army of the Rhine, Thomassin had equipped his battle surgeons and sought to standardize their techniques. Larrey, who had come to Strasbourg as surgeon-major of the military hospitals in April, 1792, termed them unhealthy and overcrowded and worked through the spring and summer to improve them. "We had few internal diseases," Larrey said, "the good constitution of the men, together with good regimen and discipline, will account for this."[19] The initial good health of the Army of the Rhine was reflected in the report by Chief Physician Lorentz in July that, out of 40,000 men, only 1,911 were hospitalized. Using Coste's standard form, Lorentz showed 953 with fevers, 280 wounded, 359 with the itch, and 319 venereals.[20]

The Army of the Rhine encountered many of the same problems that Percy faced. Lorentz and Thomassin were appalled by the lack of training of the volunteers who were enrolled as health officers, and they initiated the principle of continued studies at every opportunity. In the weeks of preparation for war, Larrey organized a school, and Thomassin required all surgeons in the Army of the Rhine to attend it. They studied anatomy and discussed questions regarding important aspects of military surgery. As Larrey recalled, "I had formed a medical society, in which everything relating to military surgery was open for discussion."[21] When the war began in earnest in the fall of 1792, Larrey continued this schooling. Now cadavers were plentiful, and whenever the army halted for a few days or weeks, operations and the study of anatomy went on.[22]

The swelling numbers of sick and wounded, however, gradually affected all the armies. By August, 1792, the Army of the North had 76,000 troops defending a line from Dunkirk to Longwy, but its hospital service, rated for only 9,000 patients, was already overloaded with 16,137 sick. The Army of the Moselle was in even worse condition. With 25,000 line troops and 35,000 reserves covering the area from Longwy east to Bitche, the Army of the Moselle's list of sick had risen from 4,000 to 11,000 when Percy took over as consulting surgeon of both armies on August 10. In the best condition was the Army of the Rhine, now composed of two corps totaling 96,000 men plus 10,000 reserves, covering the line from Mayence to Porentruy. But even its hospital facilities were strained. There were 13,000 sick being cared for by a hospital service designed for 9,600.[23]

The Prussians, starting the campaign of 1792 late, began entering France on August 19. The Duke of Brunswick followed ordinary rules of campaigning by advancing, then halting until six days' bread had been baked, and then advancing again. Before these methodical professional movements, the raw French units fell back steadily. Longwy fell, then Verdun, and the road to Paris was open. At Valmy on September 20, where the Prussians were checked by the revolutionary armies, battle casualties were only about 300 for the French and less than 200 for the Prussians, but dysentery took a frightful toll in both armies.[24] As the Prussian army retired northward, the overtaxed medical service of General Dumouriez's army could not serve the wounded plus those stricken with dysentery. Also, ophthalmia was spreading rapidly among the French troops, its outbreak coinciding with the first frost.[25]

The new National Convention, which had convened on September 22, sent "representatives on mission" to help deal with the condition of the armies. By September 24, three of them had joined the Army of the North. Ignoring the military medical officers and wielding their political powers, they took over and set up "hospitals" in confiscated buildings at Chateau-Thierry and at Sainte-Menehould. On October 7 they reported to the Convention: "Having observed that the beds of the wounded were composed only of heaps of straw, we could not conceive such thoughtlessness, and we required the municipality of Sainte-Menehould to furnish without compensation twenty-four mattresses from among its citizens who have several of them upon their beds."[26]

The nonmedical representatives of the Convention believed that energy and activity could overcome complex and overwhelming medical problems. The shortage of hospital facilities was acute in the fall of 1792, and churches, convents, and monasteries were often the first places thought of for housing the sick and wounded. As the representatives on mission from the Convention fanned out over France, they tended to share the ideas expressed by Lazare Carnot in his October 20, 1792 report: "One of the most important of our tasks, we expect, will be the founding of a military hospital; the only one that exists here, under that name, is only a sort of gloomy shelter, without equipment and without space . . . . Our proposal is to locate the hospital in one of the nationalized buildings, occupied heretofore by monks; some beds are there, and few changes will have to be made in order to receive those who will live there henceforth."[27]

The appearance of these representatives on mission immediately politicized the military medical problem. Initially the health officers had been filled with revolutionary fervor. Some 1,200 medical men had volunteered when their fellow citizens armed to defend the nation. Red, white, and blue flags flew as honors were accorded the wounded. Often the strains of the Marseillaise accompanied them through the doors of the hospital. The health officers who were providing the medical care were honored and encouraged to give every possible care to the nation's wounded sons. Military officers had done their best to commandeer whatever the physicians and surgeons required. But the political representatives of the new Convention, many of them openly contemptuous of medical men, had come to solve all problems on the spot. Asserting their powers, they intimidated the military commanders and health officers and appealed to local municipalities and Jacobin clubs. Reacting angrily, the military medical officers saw these representatives as nothing more than reincarnations of the hated old war commissioners.

Another crucial problem facing Dumouriez's army in Belgium was the lack of physicians and surgeons. Many of the health officers who had been appointed by the Minister of War had not joined the armies even by December, 1792. The critical needs of the sick and wounded in Belgium led Coste, Percy, and many other medical officers to hire local help with their own personal funds. On December 18, representatives on mission wrote to the Convention from Belgium, verifying that a number of medical men had used their own money to hire essential help and advising that all the surgeons and physicians were now "in penury" because neither salaries nor funds for hospitals had been received since October 1. The representatives begged the Convention to review the situation, adding that "it certainly seems just to us to declare that those who have been appointed to some post in moments of the greatest urgency, who are so slow in taking their places, *ipso facto* should be replaced on the spot."[28] The Council of Health, however, sent no money and responded to pleas for help by commissioning younger men who were eager to join the armies but who were inexperienced, immature, and able to answer only the most elementary medical questions.[29] Once they joined the armies, they had to be trained somehow by medical men who were already overtaxed and who needed able helpers, not students.

Coste was determined that most of the inexperienced subalterns should be put out onto the battlefield to help with the wounded. Traditional military medical practice had been to leave the wounded where they fell until the battle was over. Only then would haphazardly selected litter-bearers move out to bring those who were still alive into the field hospitals (required by law to be stationed one league away).[30] Litter-bearers so casually selected often had other interests. General Louis Charles Desaix (later killed leading an attack at Marengo) recorded his encounter with two litter-bearers who asked him to make way for a wounded man. The body was insufficiently covered and Desaix said that he "wondered at its long nose and short legs." Raising the covering, he found a dead pig—the main object of the litter-bearers' concern.[31] From a military standpoint, what usually happened when a man was wounded was far more serious. Briot, who as a battle surgeon saw it often, left a description of the procedure: "Three or four soldiers carried the wounded soldier in their arms, or on their guns, on branches, on cloaks, on coats, sometimes by means of his own clothes; a fifth carried his bag; a sixth his gun; another his shako; until six or eight soldiers left the front for every one who was struck; and a regiment which had twenty or thirty wounded soon was diminished to one-third of its strength."[32]

One of the best of Percy's innovations was his creation of a corps of stretcher-bearers who doubled as corpsmen. Old soldiers and culls from the regiments, young medical subalterns, even the able-bodied sick, were pressed into service. As Percy quipped, "In a time when the mule was a citizen, one infected with the itch could well be a corpsman."[33] Given a uniform, a knapsack of first aid materials, a pike, and a short knife, Percy's stretcher-bearers worked in pairs. Their pikes served as some protection against enemy cavalry out on the battlefield or could form the carrying arms of a litter.[34] In the fall of 1792, Percy's stretcher-bearers began moving onto the battlefield under fire, picking up the wounded as they fell, and conveying them to the mobile hospitals nearby. Once the field had been cleared, these men were expected to serve as corpsmen in the hospital area, helping physicians and surgeons in ministering to the wounded.[35]

Army field hospitals had been almost nonexistent in 1792. Therefore, to shorten the time required to get badly hurt men evacuated from the front to hospitals in the rear, Percy offered another innovation. A time lapse of from 24 to 36 hours usually occurred between the time of a wound and first medical aid, mainly because of roads clogged with vehicles of all kinds. In retreats, this was at its worst. The surgeon Jacques Cassanyes expressed his horror upon seeing how carelessly a convoy of wagons carried the wounded: "I even saw one of these unfortunate men fall out of the front of the carriage, and the wheel passed over him; the wagon drivers had neither shadow of sensitivity nor pity."[36] Percy, who had seen many retreats, wrote: "In a retreat before the enemy, there is no more frightful spectacle to be seen than the evacuation of mutilated soldiers on big wagons, from whom each jolt wrings the most piercing cries; who have to suffer from rain, from suffocating heat, or freezing cold, and who often do not have either aid or food of any sort during a long and miserable journey. Death would be a favor in this situation, and we have often heard them begging for it as a gift from Heaven."[37]

Percy's solution was to attempt to bring hospital aid closer to the battlefield by creating a mobile hospital called a *würtz*. To Percy, it was a "mobile surgical corps."[38] In his journal, he recalled his experience in trying to get his idea converted into reality: "I had proposed to our generals that my colleagues in all divisions, and especially in the vanguard, should have this kind of light and maneuverable carriage on which ten men can safely ride. I had explained the remarkable advantages for the safety, speed and improvement of medical service. They were so pleased that several such *würtz* minus the horses, were immediately put at my disposal by the artillery officers. But the horses became the stumbling block of our project. They were never refused, but such were the obstacles, pretexts and excuses that the *würtzs* were returned to the arsenal whence they had been taken . . . . Some thought that it might have been a dangerous sight to see surgeons ride, since a system full of ill-will, oppression and humiliation had long condemned them to walk and be covered with dust and dirt; they *should* walk and be miserable, otherwise, some adminis-trators said, they would become too cocky."[39]

Despite the fact that the Convention had been deluged with petitions from medical officers begging for hospital ambulances and their equipment, the Convention still had provided no funds.[40] Nevertheless, Thomassin, surgeon-in-chief of the Army of the Rhine, and Larrey joined in the creation of a light mobile ambulance similar to Percy's wagon. Each one was equipped to care for about one hundred wounded men and was staffed by four mounted surgeons.[41] Neither of these types was intended as an evacuation vehicle per se, because it was believed that the Austrians would accept Percy's proposal to give hospitals, health officers, and wounded men immunity from any military action. Although General Moreau adopted the idea, General Kray, the Austrian commander, refused to agree, and the chief value of the slow and heavy *würtz* was to bring to the battlefield a type of medical aid heretofore unavailable.[42] Briot, who was attached to one of these heavy ambulance hospitals, recorded an insight into their usefulness: "I prepared in advance everything which my colleagues and I would need for dressing two, three or four thousand wounded, sometimes an even greater number, according to estimated needs. Supplies of rags, strips of all sizes, elastic agglutinative patches, compresses of every shape and style, bandages of all sorts; all was prepared, stacked, labelled, numbered in the boxes which never left the ambulance: everything was at our fingertips when we needed it. With one eye we saw the nature of the wound; with the other, the most suitable relief."[43]

When the Army of the Rhine moved out on September 30 into the Rhineland, Larrey was assigned to Houchard's advance guard as chief surgeon. The town of Spire (Speyer) was taken quickly, and General Custine directed Houchard's force on toward Worms. During a sharp reverse at Ober-Ursel, Larrey felt the anguish of seeing his wounded left to fall into enemy hands. As he watched the light artillery quickly wheel out of danger, he conceived of a light, two-wheeled evacuation vehicle for rapidly carrying battle casualties to the rear. With Houchard's approval and the ingenuity of the chief quartermaster, Villemanzy, several of these light, two-wheeled carriages were constructed and placed in service under Larrey's direction.[44] Briot, who was assigned to these "flying ambulances" when the Army of the Moselle was united with the Army of the Rhine, has left the best description: "When I was attached to the flying ambulances, we usually had from twenty to twenty-five suspended carriages, covered and with comfortably lined interiors; in each one two patients could lie down comfortably .... Four could get in if their wounds did not require them to lie down. This carriage hitched to a single horse, took the wounded to the nearest hospital and sometimes made four, five, or six trips a day. Only those who could not walk were put in the carriages."[45]

The Army of the North did not have even this small beginning of light evacuation vehicles. An unknown painter of the battle of Jemappes (November 6, 1792) depicted a wagon quite like the American Conestoga, jammed with wounded, being laboriously pulled to the rear by straining men and horses.[46] Five days after Jemappes, the National Convention finally recognized that the evacuation problem had not been solved by the mobile hospitals. It appropriated 100,000 livres to the War Minister, who ordered construction of springed carriages for the transport of sick and wounded. Designed to carry three patients on each side, these four-wheeled wagons were to be drawn by four horses and supplied to the armies on the basis of one for each 1,000 effective troops.[47] The fine performance, however, of the "flying ambulance" improvised by Larrey soon forced a reconsideration of the Convention's design. When Custine's overextended position in Germany forced the Army of the Rhine to begin retreating in March, 1793, the flying ambulances performed an evacuation service so remarkable that Larrey was shortly summoned to Paris to direct the design and construction of similar vehicles for all of the armies.[48]

In the meantime, a contest with a 2,000-livre prize was announced by the War Ministry for the best design of an evacuation vehicle similar to Larrey's improvised carriage. However, the specifications for the vehicle were totally unrealistic. It was to be "light and solid," able to hold four prone sick men or "a greater number half-crouching," but the vehicle was to be no taller than a man's height and "always roomy." It was to carry every means of satisfying a patient's needs but simply constructed and easy to repair. The vehicle was to be planned so as to protect the passengers from insects, rain, heat, and cold but designed so as not to impede the flow of fresh air and the access of light. Finally, it was to be versatile; when there were no patients to transport, the vehicle had to be useful "for other things."[49]

The delay this contest entailed meant that the ambulance service was not even ready for the fall campaign of 1793. At Wattignies (October 16–18), four-wheeled covered wagons were crammed indiscriminately with sick and wounded men, and the surgeons complained bitterly of wagons "more likely to aggravate the condition of the wounded than to comfort them."[50] Indeed, able-bodied troops often refused to ride in wagons designated to transport them, preferring to walk.[51] After repeated delays, two designs for evacuation vehicles were published by the War

Ministry very late in 1793, but both were ultimately rejected. The Great Committee of Public Safety ordered the construction of a few carriages which were composites of various designs that had been submitted but the result was dismal. What emerged from the wagon-builder's shop was remarkably like Percy's *würtz*, "a true hospital ambulance . . . which required eight horses to pull it."[52] The mouse, when built to government specifications, had turned into an elephant! During all this delay, the military medical men in the field had to continue to improvise and requisition light carriages and wagons filled with straw and furnished with confiscated bedding.

During winter quarters after the campaign of 1792, an epidemic illness, probably influenza, broke out in the Army of the Rhine.[53] The winter was a rainy one; the armies were fatigued and lacking in clothes and boots. Food was usually scarce and uniformly bad. Joliclerc, a volunteer of 1792, wrote: "One must be content with his bread which is not good, and with his half-pound of meat off a rotten carcass that the dogs would not eat."[54] Another volunteer complained: "Twenty ounces of bread, which is worse than congealed oats, with a half-pound of meat with which one can no more make soup than with a stick of wood."[55] Percy himself asserted that "many times the military surgeons had to kill their horses to make soup for the wounded, who would have died without that wise precaution."[56] The privations suffered by the armies during the winter and early spring of 1793 jammed the hospitals with sick men. The Army of the North was so epidemic-ridden that the frontier between France and Belgium was closed by roadblocks in an effort to control the spread of disease.[57]

Meanwhile, from the reports of medical men, hospital administrators, and representatives on mission during the period from the fall of 1792 to the spring of 1793, the pattern of wartime ailments and the magnitude of the medical emergency had begun to emerge. Three medical inspectors, Bertrand Pelletier, Claude Boyer, and Pierre Groffier, sent in repeated pleas for money, medicines, and supplies for the hospitals of the north.

At Tournai on December 10, 1792, the hospital rated for 50 patients had 145 jammed within its walls. The hospital administrator was a 21 year old named Clement. The protégé of a wealthy uncle, he was found to be "too young and ignorant." Dismissed for "negligence and incompetence," Clement was replaced by a veteran local physician.[58] The report by Pelletier, Boyer, and Groffier, dated December 28, on the ambulance hospitals at Saint Jean and at Carmes included the standard pharmacy inventory of drugs and supplies. The column headed "superfluous" is virtually empty while the "needed" column is almost completely filled, with "urgently" handwritten across the top. The hospital at Saint Jean (rated for 100) had 144 wounded and no place near to which they could be evacuated. The latrines were termed "insufficient, unhealthy and improper," the linens "bad," and the surgical equipment "incomplete." Only one surgeon aide-major commanded nine surgeons and four apothecaries, and Boyer remarked that "the practice of the aide-major is neither enlightened nor followed" by his subordinates.[59]

From Landrécy on January 2, 1793, Boyer reported that the town had offered them a church and a convent for hospital facilities. Complaining that the church was filthy, humid, and poorly ventilated, he told the Council of Health: "We are short of medicines; especially do we need quinine and good quality wine, which is better than topicals for cleaning wounds."[60] The normal garrison at Dunkirk had been small, and the military medical facilities limited. By November 26, 1792, there were over 8,000 men concentrated there, and a total of 303 sick and wounded had overflowed its capacity. The medical inspectors on January 2, 1793, suggested seizure of the big Recollets convent to ease the pressure, recommending that the military hospitals keep the fever patients and send all others to the Recollets. However, by June the Recollets was full, and the military hospital was reporting 350 patients.[61]

From the area around Maubeuge, the medical inspectors continued to relay to Paris details of complaints of people who had not been paid and demands of others for indemnity. One enterprising young ambulance surgeon requested a promotion, saying, "You can forget about my back pay."[62] Some hospital employees had not been paid in eighteen months, and practically all were "on starvation rations." The hospitals were dilapidated and without pharmacists, and the former religious orders were uncooperative. The three inspectors admitted that some of this resistance was justified by the way they had been treated but affirmed that "it is still essential to reform these enterprises in order to put all hospitals under a uniform system." They found the ambulance hospitals overloaded and underequipped: "the linen for bandaging is of mediocre quality, there are no roller-bandages at all, and the lint for stuffing wounds is of very bad quality."[63] The Maubeuge hospital itself was a converted chateau with three floors, usually equipped and staffed for 60 sick out of a garrison of 1,600. In December, 1792, it held 300 patients and the mortality rate had been nearly one in four. The report concluded: "The pharmacy is run by the local apothecary's assistant and the books do not conform to the rules of the Health Service. The stairs are difficult to climb and the latrines are improperly installed. There are now 389 patients in this hospital which is rated for only 60; 258 with fevers and 100 wounded. The main fevers are catarrhal, bilious, simple or putrid. Many of the wounded are badly mutilated."[64]

At Brussels, on January 17, the three medical inspectors promptly suspended the administrator of the St. Elizabeth hospital for incompetence. In this converted convent, there were 1,116 patients, and the agents reported that "the hospital had no fresh air, not enough latrines, not enough water and is badly overcrowded. We are now practically out of medicinals, even though they requested them over three months ago."[65] Appended to this report was a detailed inventory of medicines and drugs. There were only two items in the entire hospital pharmacy considered surplus: 14 ounces of antimony and 16 ounces of sulphur. From a long list of 158 different items,[66] the following common ingredients indicate the severity of the shortage.

Medicinal	[Often used for]	On hand	Needed
Soda	[widely used in prescriptions]	8 #	80 #
Species pectorales	[prescription bases]	12 #	200 #
Wine	[wounds]	0 #	360 #
Olive oil	[abscesses, wounds]	66 #	140 #
Lead oxide	[burns]	4 #	20 #
Calx	[antiseptic or stimulant]	0 #	15 #
Muriatic acid	[ophthalmia]	0 #	6 #
Senna	[a cathartic]	3 #	80 #
Guaicum	[antivenereal]	0 #	6 #
Mercury (all types)	[antivenereal]	0 #	8 #
Rhubarb	[hospital gangrene]	1 #	8 #
Rhubarb (pulverized)	[hospital gangrene]	2 #	20 #
Ipecacuanha	[dysentery]	1 oz.	6 #
Laudanum	[dysentery]	3 oz.	3 #
Iron sulfide	[the itch]	0 #	1 #
Zinc sulfide	[the itch]	0 #	8 #

Wartime hospital diseases were both mysterious and devastating. In December, 1792, great numbers of men were dying in the hospitals around Cambrai from an unknown ailment. In an attempt to identify it, the Executive Council in Paris had to call upon the Minister of War to leave at once for Cambrai, taking Fourcroy and Roussillon with him in the capacity of medical specialists.[67]

Representatives of the Convention inspected hospitals near the armies but their reports were not always accurate. On January 19, 1793, Gossuin and Camus reported the Louvain hospital "very well tended," possibly because it was being supervised by a political agent of the Executive Council. From Strasbourg, Couturier wrote vaguely on February 8 of "a number of abuses to redress," while Dubois-Crancé wrote cryptically of "the spirit of insubordination in the hospitals."[68] Deville attempted to gloss over the inadequacies of the hospitals of Soissons, Laon, and Sedan by utilizing negative expressions: "Food and supplies are not lacking . . . but the linen is not good, and there is not a great number of attendants."[69] At the same time that one representative was implying that there were no field hospitals with the Army of the North and charging that soldiers had to go sixty leagues to be treated, another was reporting the heroism of a wounded corporal who walked "half a league" to a mobile hospital to be treated.[70]

As the French armies moved further into Belgium and Germany, they found that hospital facilities became even worse. At Liège, men in the lice-ridden hospital "captured these vermin by the handful," and the representatives on mission found most of the sick lying on the floor, without mattresses or blankets. On December 8, they reported that, having appealed to the town government in vain, they appeared before the "Friends of Liberty and Equality," the local Jacobin club. "We gave them the picture of the state in which we found our wounded; and we see today that they are carrying mattresses and blankets through the door of the hospital."[71] Despite such isolated efforts, however, conditions prevailing in the hospitals continued to be uniformly bad. At Cologne in December, for example, "the men lay on pallets or on the ground, without sheets, under the worst coverings, *full of lice* . . . . "[72]

Out of this welter of reports, conflicting, sometimes exaggerated, but increasingly ominous, by both medical and political observers, a picture emerged of inadequate medical facilities, poor equipment, crowded conditions, and an acute shortage of medicines and medical men. The mass armies created by revolutionary France were on the offensive against the enemy, but their sicknesses and wounds were beginning to overwhelm the medical service.

Health officers were in short supply in the early months of 1793 for a variety of reasons. Out of 1,400 enrolled in 1792, over 600 had perished on the battlefield or from disease. Others were wounded or otherwise disabled.[73] Many simply left for home—they had volunteered to care for the defenders of the nation, and the defenders were now in Belgium and Germany. Without equipment and medicines, without pay for months, many saw nothing to do but to go home and support their families. Some medical men had been dismissed for obvious incompetency, but the swiftly developing antagonism between the representatives on mission and the medical service produced even more dismissals. Although "incompetence" was the reason given in reports to Paris, in many cases the representatives on mission could have more honestly worded it "insubordination" or "personal vendetta." As the medical officers continued to resent, resist, and impede the expanding assertions of medical authority by the political representatives, the remaining health officers were subject to new harassment. Local Jacobins denounced their lack of patriotism or attacked them as traitors for continuing to wear their gold-decorated uniforms. Consequently even more left the service and some even emigrated.[74]

By March, 1793, when the French armies were retreating before the Austro-Prussian advance in the Low Countries and along the Rhine, the rising tide of sick and wounded revealed how critically short was the supply of military medical men. Levasseur wrote to the Convention from Metz about the overcrowded hospitals and the lack of medical men, advising that "the neighboring departments, although plagued by a shortage of health officers, have drafted theirs to send them to us."[75] The representatives on mission, confronted with a new crisis, began reporting "a growing number of desertions" among health officers. One reported from Valenciennes on March 9 on "the bad conduct of a great number of health officers near the armies of the North and of the Ardennes . . . ."[76] Two days later, Camus and Treilhard from Louvain charged that "no health officers remained at Liège to look after the needs of the sick."[77] The representatives on mission had contributed to the critical scarcity of medical men by their harassment of them and their decision-making in medical matters. Simply reporting the number of dead or disabled medical men and reminding the Convention that those who survived had little equipment, few medicines, and no pay since October, 1792, was too risky an explanation. So the easiest way to explain why the defenders of the nation went uncared for was to blame the medical service and report a wave of "desertions."

As the retreat of the French armies became a rout, the medical service was attacked more vigorously than ever. A representative on mission, Delacroix, described an action near Louvain on March 21 and charged: "The army could have held much longer but for the cowardice of the stretcher-bearers who, by their flight, threw it into disorder and spread alarm in one segment of our troops."[78] Bézard and Thibault, writing to the Convention from Chantilly, sounded an increasingly common complaint. They accused physicians of permitting troops infected with trench-foot to loiter in the hospitals when they were needed to stem the enemy advance. They told the Convention that "those soldiers, attacked by *a simple skin disease*, think they are unable to bear arms and serve their country." Neither was a physician but they asserted that "the season is not at all favorable for the treatment of this disease and, if you will announce that all who have it are required to rejoin the colors, you will have 40,000 men in fighting condition immediately."[79]

As the French armies began to collapse, and battle after battle was lost, no one wanted to admit that republican citizen-soldiers could be so badly defeated by the minions of tyrants. When the defenders of the nation broke and ran, medical corpsmen and stretcher-bearers could take the blame. In a time when anyone could practice medicine, the representatives on mission diagnosed the shortage of effective troops. It was not due to the terrible battle casualties that had been suffered nor to the disabling diseases affecting the foot soldier—it was the fault of the military physicians! The zeal and fanaticism of the political representatives, when heightened by the panic of seeing the armies routed and reeling drunkenly back into France, became an intolerable burden for medical men at a time when their best services were desperately needed.

A tremendous additional strain upon the medical service was the large number of troops infected with venereal diseases. Many women and girls, inspired by the Revolution, had disguised themselves as men and joined the armies despite the strict rules and severe penalties of the April 30, 1792, Decree on Women with the Armies.[80] Larrey insisted that he knew one woman in the Army of the Rhine "whose conduct was perfectly regular and who had taken such good precautions that none of her comrades had ever suspected."[81] Some women did distinguish themselves, such as Catherine Pochelat, a Paris volunteer of 1792, cited for heroism at Jemappes as a gun-server in General Dampierre's artillery, or Marie Schelling, who collected six sabre wounds and the nickname of "the sergeant of Jemappes." Others, of very doubtful value, were women organized into battalions by some eager Jacobins, who sent "these new amazons" to the front.[82] Combined with the regular horde of camp followers, such women infected the troops and filled the hospitals with them. In the retreat, these women clogged the roads ahead of the retiring army. Officers and medical men alike pleaded with the Convention to do something about "the scourge of women and girls who follow the army."[83] One representative on mission demanded, "Make the armies chase off these damned women who lose us more soldiers than muskets, cannon, and bayonets."[84] Another reported that, on the retreat from Belgium in April, 1793, the women "formed a second army."[85]

Scattered among this horde of fleeing women were many deserting stretcher-bearers, hangers-on, and those unfit troops who were the first to panic and flee, crying "Every man for himself."[86] They flooded the reserve hospitals, and Carnot estimated that there were "50,000 sick, syphilitic, epileptic, malingerers of all sorts" in the retreat.[87] They pillaged the hospitals at Liège, and at Aix-la-Chapelle in March, 1793, and carried off all the mattresses and coverings.[88] The representatives on mission continued to report the steady disappearance of hospital staffs and the growing demoralization of hospital services.[89] Beffroy wrote from Cambrai to the Convention that everything was disorganized and that the army lacked everything. Prieur de la Marne, with the army near La Rochelle, told the same story. After General Dumouriez deserted in April, Carra summarized the condition of the Army of the North on the Saumur River: "Nobody knows the general movement of the troops which make up the army; no general staff, no adjutant generals, no officers of supply, forage, hospitals, etc."[90]

The military medical service that had been improvised in 1792 fell apart rapidly in the early spring of 1793. The roads leading back into France from Belgium and the Rhineland were littered with dead horses and broken or mired hospital wagons. Fleeing health officers carried away their bags of equipment or left them behind to be broken open and scattered by pillagers. The medical service was paralyzed by a lack of funds. Salaries were months in arrears despite the Convention's promises, and many medical men had simply gone home rather than starve. Nor did the Convention supply the money necessary to operate and supply the military hospitals. Supplies of bedding, bandages, and medicines were seriously depleted. The military hospitals were understaffed and choked with sick and wounded. The reserve hospitals in the towns and communes were also paralyzed by a lack of staff, an acute shortage of funds, the religious controversy, and the flood of battle casualties and the sick. Typhus and cholera appeared and raced through the horribly overcrowded hospital facilities, taking a terrible toll of health officers as well as of troops.

War, desertion, and disease had taken off nearly three-fourths of the medical men enrolled since 1792. With the medical schools abolished, no newly trained replacements could be foreseen. The Convention's representatives on mission, having contributed significantly to the shattered morale of the medical service, now blamed it not only for failing to do the impossible but for the military disaster as well. It was apparent by the end of the spring of 1793 that, if hospital services were to be available, if sufficient physicians and surgeons were to be had, and if adequate medical supplies and transport were to be acquired, new and extraordinary measures would have to be taken.

NOTES

1. Coste dossier, carton 205/1, Val-de-Grâce; Dufresnoy dossier, carton 207/3, ibid.; Gorcy dossier, carton 209/1, ibid.; Lorentz dossier, carton 209/1, ibid.; Rieux and Hassenforder, *Histoire*, p.125.

2. Saucerotte dossier, carton 213, Val-de-Grâce; Parmentier dossier, ·carton 211, ibid.; Percy dossier, carton 211 bis, ibid.; Rapports, carton 22, Arch. hist. Service de Santé; Rieux and Hassenforder, *Histoire*, p.125.

3. Coste dossier, carton 205/1, Val-de-Grâce. Folio B contains the letters written by George Washington and Voltaire and the honorary degree awarded by the University of Pennsylvania on December 23, 1782.

4. This *Instruction* by the Committee of Health is in Coste dossier, folio D, carton 205/1, Val-de-Grâce.

5. Armées du Nord, carton 25, Arch. hist. Service de Santé.

6. Ibid.

7. Ibid.

8. Rapports aux inspecteurs-généraux, folio 1, carton 21, ibid.

9. Ibid.

10. Report of the Committee of Health, Acq. fran. 3: 21a, folio D, p.5, Archives nationales.

11. Larrey, *Memoirs* 1: 80, 104; Thompson, *Surgical Instruments*, pp.15, 22.

12. Laurent, *Percy*, pp.344–48.

13. Phipps, *Armies of the First Republic* 1: 16.

14. Cabanès, *Chirurgiens et blessés*, pp.311–12.

15. Briot, *Chirurgie militaire*, p.339.

16. Lafont-Gouzi, *Matériaux*, p.9.

17. Briot, *Chirurgie militaire*, p.371.

18. Cabanès, *Chirurgiens et blessés*, p.319. Italics of Cabanès.

19. Larrey, *Memoirs* 1: 31.

20. Conseil de Santé, carton 13, Arch. hist. Service de Santé; Armées du Rhin, carton 29, ibid.

21. Larrey, *Memoirs* 1: 22.

22. J. Chalmers Da Costa, "Baron Larrey: A Sketch," *Johns Hopkins Hospital Bulletin* 17: 200–1; Triaire, *Larrey*, p.51.

23. Samuel F. Scott, "The Regeneration of the Line Army during the French Revolution," *Journal of Modern History* 42: 321–23; Ganges, *Représentants du peuple* 1: 150–51.

24. Phipps, *Armies of the First Republic* 2: 27; Hoffman Nickerson, *The Armed Horde, 1793–1939: A Study in the Rise, Survival, and Decline*

of the Mass Army (New York, 1940), pp.77—78.

25. Lafont-Gouzi, *Matériaux*, p.39. This convinced Lafont-Gouzi that ophthalmia (probably conjunctivitis) was caused by changes in temperature.

26. Aulard, *Recueil des actes* 1: 67, 108—9.

27. Ibid., 1: 173.

28. Cabanès, *Chirurgiens et blessés*, p.338.

29. Larrey, *Memoirs* 1: 22.

30. Ibid., 1: 23; Garrison, *Notes*, p.165.

31. Phipps, *Armies of the First Republic* 2: 65.

32. Briot, *Chirurgie militaire*, p.400.

33. Laurent, *Percy*, p.378.

34. Cabanès, *Chirurgiens et blessés*, p.344. The uniform (rarely worn) was a short coat of brown linen with a red collar and lapels, brown pants with red stripes down the sides, red vest, and a round hat with a stripe of gold braid and decorated with colored plumes.

35. Briot, *Chirurgie militaire*, p.401; Laignel-Lavastine, *Histoire générale* 3: 7; Triaire, "Tactique sanitaire," *Caducée* 2: 158.

36. Vidal, "Documents inédits," *Révolution française* 16: 462.

37. Laurent, *Percy*, p.196.

38. Percy dossier, carton 211 bis, Val-de-Grâce. The origin of this term is obscure but it probably was coined by Prussians from the German word *würze* (seasoning, spices, aromatic herbs). See *Deutsches Wörterbuch von Jacob Grimm und Wilhelm Grimm* (Leipzig, 1960), 14, part 2, 2328. Since eighteenth-century medicines consisted principally of spices and herbs, these huge medicine-carrying wagons most likely received this appellation from the Prussians who adopted them in their own military medical system after the campaign of 1792. See Triaire, "Tactique sanitaire," *Caducée* 2: 158.

39. Percy, *Journal*, p.3.

40. Armées du Nord, carton 25, Arch. hist. Service de Santé, is filled with such pleas.

41. Laurent, *Percy*, pp.197—99; Triaire, *Larrey*, p.26.

42. Laurent, *Percy*, pp.197—99.

43. Briot, *Chirurgie militaire*, pp.380—81.

44. Larrey, *Memoirs* 1: 22—23; Triaire, *Larrey*, pp.25—29; Laignel-Lavastine, *Histoire générale* 3: 7.

45. Briot, *Chirurgie militaire*, pp.404—5. Larrey's early biographer, Triaire (*Larrey*, p.29), described the "flying ambulance" in terms that confuse it with the light hospital that Larrey and Thomassin created. Garrison, *Notes*, p.165, refers to "light, closed two-wheelers carrying two wounded men each, drawn by two horses. . . ." Briot, André Soubiran, *Baron Larrey*, pp.48ff., and Singer, *Short History*, p.184, correctly refer to "a light one-horse vehicle which could remove casualties quickly from

quite near the fighting line," and these descriptions tally with that in Larrey's *Memoirs* 1: 28ff.

46. Reproduced in Cabanès, *Chirurgiens et blessés*, p.363.

47. Bottet, "Le passé," *Caducée* 5:151.

48. Triaire, "Tactique sanitaire," ibid., 2: 157—58; Cabanès, *Chirurgiens et blessés*, p.376.

49. Cabanès, *Chirurgiens et blessés*, p.376—77.

50. Ibid., pp.362—65. Canal boats were sometimes used when the armies were in the Low Countries but in a retreat they were useless. See M. Ferron, "Le service de santé des armées françaises et les évacuations par eau de 1743 à 1832," *Archives de médecine et pharmacie militaire* 59: 455—56.

51. Aulard, *Recueil des actes* 6: 151.

52. Cabanès, *Chirurgiens et blessés*, pp.379—80.

53. Larrey, *Memoirs* 1: 34. The training of health officers was continued during winter quarters of 1792—93. Courses were set up at the Strasbourg hospital that required them to take lessons in operating medicine, anatomy, and diagnosis.

54. Quoted in Phipps, *Armies of the First Republic* 2: 33.

55. Quoted in Cabanès *Chirurgiens et blessés*, p.314.

56. Percy dossier, carton 211 bis, Val-de-Grâce.

57. Aulard, *Recueil des actes* 4: 253.

58. Armées du Nord, carton 25, Arch. hist. Service de Santé.

59. Ibid.

60. Ibid.

61. Ibid.; L. Lemaire, *Historique de l'hôpital militaire de Dunkerque* (Paris, 1936), pp.891—93.

62. Corps de Santé rapports, carton 24, Arch. hist. Service de Santé.

63. Armées du Nord, carton 25, ibid.

64. Ibid.

65. Armées de la Moselle, carton 28, ibid.

66. Armées du Nord, carton 25, ibid.

67. Aulard, *Recueil des actes* 1: 343.

68. Ibid., 1: 487; 2: 76; 4: 305.

69. Ganges, *Représentants du peuple* 2: 201.

70. Ibid. 1: 409.

71. Cabanès, *Chirurgiens et blessés*, p.320; Aulard, *Recueil des actes* 1: 304—5.

72. Cabanès, *Chirurgiens et blessés*, p.320. Italics of Cabanès.

73. Dora Weiner, "French Doctors Face War, 1792—1815," in *From the Ancien Régime to the Popular Front*, ed. C. K. Warner (New York, 1969), p.58; Laignel-Lavastine, *Histoire générale* 2: 449.

74. Aulard, *Recueil des actes* 1: 412; 2:318; Ganges, *Représentants du peuple* 1: 301.

75. Aulard, *Recueil des actes* 5: 17—18.

76. Ibid., 2: 318; 4: 305.

77. Ibid., 2: 338.

78. Ibid., 2: 446.

79. Ibid., 3: 137. Italics mine.

80. Ganges, *Représentants du peuple* 3: 575–76. The decree required explusion of all "useless" women from the armies. Four washerwomen were allowed for each battalion; generals of divisions could authorize women to deliver food or supplies, but all women had to wear a distinctive mark to show their authorized status. Women found serving in the ranks were to be sent home, being given five sous per mile for expenses. The penalty for coming back was prison (for the first offense); a second offense required that a returning woman be shot.

81. Triaire, *Larrey*, p.32.

82. Aulard, *Recueil des actes* 3: 529; 5: 315–16, 372; Ganges, *Représentants de peuple* 3: 62–64.

83. Aulard, *Recueil des actes* 3: 287; 4: 234.

84. Ibid., 3: 137.

85. Ganges, *Représentants du peuple* 3: 576.

86. Aulard, *Recueil des actes* 4: 110; Nickerson, *Armed Horde*, p.75.

87. Aulard, *Recueil des actes* 5: 220.

88. Ibid., 2: 444.

89. Ibid., 4: 305; 5: 17–18.

90. Ibid., 3: 136; 4: 44, 516.

Chapter Six

THE CRISIS OF 1793

On March 18, 1793, the retreating Army of the North was defeated by the Austrians at Neerwinden and again on the 21st at Louvain. General Custine's Army of the Rhine abandoned the left bank of that river on March 28, falling back upon Landau and leaving Mayence to a Prussian siege. General Dumouriez, commanding the reeling Army of the North, negotiated an armistice; then suddenly, on April 5, deserted to the enemy. The next day, to cope with domestic disorder and the grave war emergency, the Convention created the first Committee of Public Safety, headed by Danton. Soon the Austrians under Prince Coburg were besieging Condé and Valenciennes in the north of France. When Cambrai was left unprotected by the retreating French army on May 23, Paris was extremely vulnerable to any swift move southward by the enemy. The National Convention's effort of February 24 to reinforce its collapsing armies with a conscription of 300,000 men had met with resistance from the outset. When 82 representatives were commissioned on March 9 to enforce this levy, the Convention was confronted with a serious threat from another direction—the West. The Vendée rose in revolt, and by March 14 what was to be a prolonged and bloody civil war was underway.

The Committee of Public Safety, in decreeing an army to suppress the revolt, ordered the Minister of War to establish "in that army both mobile and fixed hospitals" and to "send health officers and employees in sufficient number . . . ."[1] But the already alarming shortage of medical men and facilities precluded any such action. Besides, the Jacobins in the Vendée had already begun to convert into prisons most of the buildings which might have been used for hospitals. The bitter and bloody nature of the struggle in the Vendée did not encourage the establishment of a medical service. Wounded men were put out of their misery or just left to die, and when the prisons that were secure were full, it became easier to shoot captured rebels and leave them lying by the roadsides.[2] Félix, a national commissioner with the Army of the West, reported on September 14, 1793, that "eight hundred scoundrels have been killed and the roads are covered with their hideous bodies."[3] General Westermann informed the Convention, "I have not a single prisoner with which to reproach myself. I have wiped out all . . . . The roads are strewn with corpses . . . . We take no prisoners at all . . . . "[4] After the rebel rout at Le Mans on December 13, hundreds were shot as they fled along the roads to Laval and Alençon. In December and January, the representative Francastel had between fifteen hundred and two thousand rebels executed near Angers.[5] What was principally needed in the Vendée was a burial squad, not a medical service.

The "no-quarter" policy adopted by both government and rebel forces in the Vendée soon shifted the Convention's concern from a lack of hospitals to a fear of epidemics. Reports continued to pour in concerning vast numbers of cadavers lying in the open along the roads of the Vendée and even of many poorly interred bodies on the northern frontier. Guyton de Morveau and Fourcroy were asked to study and report the best means of disposing of bodies, uninterred or carelessly buried, which could cause epidemics.[6] Except for the order of May 4, 1793, to create a medical service for the army in the Vendée, the Committee of Public Safety was silent on the subject thereafter. If no one attempted to implement that decree, it was partly due to an acute lack of medical personnel and partly due to the savage nature of the war that was fought in the Vendée. Nowhere else were the consequences of a lack of the humane work of hospitals and medical men more evident: "Thousands of rebels and rebel suspects were shot, guillotined, or drowned, making some of the towns of the West veritable charnel houses. The stench of the putrescent corpses . . . thinly buried on the outskirts of Nantes, infected the western quarters of the city; dogs dragged human flesh through the streets; and, naturally enough, an epidemic of cholera broke out."[7]

With the evident failure of Danton's peace policy, the power struggle between Jacobins and Girondins had intensified. The Jacobins lost control of Marseilles on April 29, and Lyon rose in revolt, with severe street fighting on May 29. However, the Jacobins won political power in the Convention on June 2 when the Paris sections forced the Convention to arrest 29 Girondin deputies, though some of these proscribed Girondins managed to flee and organize a new civil war. At Lyon, Marseilles, and Toulon, Jacobins were guillotined or hanged. So few troops were available to the Convention that food shipments to Paris were not protected, the capital was vulnerable to the rebels of the Vendée, and the revolts of the south could not be quickly suppressed. By July, it appeared that France was disintegrating. The rebels of Lyon had appealed to the Sardinians for help, and Marseilles and Toulon had called for British assistance. The armies of the Alps and of Italy were almost cut off from behind. The Spanish had breached the French defenses in the Pyrenees and were penetrating southern France.[8]

On April 6, when the Committee of Public Safety was created, the Convention had also dispatched one of its members, the physician René Levasseur, as a deputy on mission to the disintegrating Army of the North, and had armed him with extraordinary powers. The critical situation that France continued to face prompted Fabre l'Eglantine and Barère to propose the creation of additional agents, deputies assigned to the various armies and given powers similar to Levasseur's. David proposed a costume (a bandolier, a sword, and a tricolored hat plume) and Thuriot moved that these agents be called "representatives of the people." Accordingly, the Convention designated Carnot, Gasparin, Bries, Roux-Fazillac, Duquesnoy, Dubois-Dubay, Duhem, and Delbrel to join the armies of the North and of the Ardennes at once. As the crisis of 1793 deepened, other deputies were sent out, such as the surgeon Jacques Cassanyes of Perpignan who was assigned to the armies of the Pyrenees especially to try to reorganize the medical service there.[9]

These new representatives of the Convention found the problems of the armies complicated and intensified by rivalries between the various civilian agents of the government and by sharp conflicts of authority between these civilian agents, the military officers, and the medical men. There were representatives on mission, agents of the various government ministries, agents for the eleven armies and the eighty-three departments, and agents for Paris and other towns. Requisitioning for a multitude of purposes in the spring and summer of 1793, these agents "roamed the length and breadth of the country, finding their supplies wherever they could, trying to outwit each other, disregarding, because of the pressure behind them, the needs of the country."[10]

The agents sent out by the Provisional Executive Council, especially from the War Ministry, had been given many duties, including visiting the hospitals and making monthly reports of any abuses or neglect.[11] As late as July 10, a dispatch from Laurent, Ferry, and Ruamps, on mission with the Army of the Rhine, underscored the problem of having numerous agents with overlapping jurisdictions: "This commissioner [Valentin Probst] is the sixth who has presented himself to us in this army since the middle of May. It seems that the Minister of War does not know how to do anything except by extraordinary agents, and that he is not satisfied with the multitude of those who the Republic pays well for various functions but he wants to add others under more or less absurd pretexts."[12]

Because the Girondins in the Convention deliberately sent Jacobin deputies on mission in order to weaken their opposition, Levasseur, an implacable foe of the Girondins, had been the first named. The group of representatives that followed him out of Paris contained other Jacobins noted for their republican zeal. The great urgency of their missions was indicated by the Convention's April 30 decree which described their powers as "unlimited."[13] Nevertheless, the Jacobin representatives met with stout opposition. "More than once," Lefebvre noted, "they encountered the violent anger of local authorities who had remained Girondins or who styled themselves as such."[14] Levasseur and Anthoine, his companion on a mission to the Army of the Moselle, were arrested in May by authorities of the town of Nancy. At Orléans, the deputies on mission were received with great hostility and one of their number, Léonard Bourdon, was attacked and wounded.[15]

As open hostility and violence met the representatives on mission, the Girondin policy of sending out Jacobins began to backfire. In the provinces, pressed by the Jacobin clubs, the administrative bodies had also created their own committees of public safety to mobilize resources against invasion and to institute severe security measures. The comprehensive instructions to representatives on mission, issued by the Committee of Public Safety on May 6, 1793, not only formally invested them with "unlimited powers," but spelled out their responsibilities in detail. These instructions allowed the Jacobin representatives a free hand in selecting members of the local committees of public safety, and they naturally chose members of the Jacobin clubs. Moving swiftly, the Jacobins smashed at their enemies by purging the provincial administrations and by arresting "suspects." They then turned their attention to restoring the ability of the armies to resist the invading enemy by levying taxes and prescribing requisitions.[16]

Although the military medical service was dissolving in the spring and summer of 1793, military physicians and surgeons angrily resented the way Jacobin political agents were "meddling" in the medical profession. Men like Percy remembered the cooperation, appreciation, and courteous treatment that army officers had given the medical men in 1792 when a military medical service had had to be improvised.[17] Therefore it was a profound shock to many of them when representatives of the Convention appeared, using their unlimited powers. That they confiscated mattresses, beds, linens, instruments, and other equipment for the use of the medical service was acceptable, but these representatives also insisted upon examining the condition of the field hospitals, determining the quality of the administration, and, worst of all, inquiring about the competence of medical men. Under their instructions, the representatives also checked on sanitary conditions in hospital rooms and corridors, pharmacies, kitchens, and bakeries. They inspected the nursing service, forcing both supply and medical officers to remedy every deficiency or face the consequences. Empowered to issue "the necessary orders to procure to the wounded and to the sick all the aid which their situation requires,"[18] the representatives on mission energetically undertook to try to hold the military medical service together.

The same problems that had plagued the medical services in the northern armies during 1792 also existed in the south of France in early 1793. Larrey, who had been called to Paris in March to organize flying ambulances for all of the armies, in April was named chief surgeon of the army that was being raised to subdue the rebel Paoli on Corsica. He turned over the task of administering the contest for ambulance designs to the Academy of Sciences, and the project soon languished amid the bureaucratic confusion of Paris.[19] The revolt of Toulon and Marseilles canceled the Corsican expedition, however, and the unexpected fighting in southern France made the organization of medical services there imperative. The new Inspector of Hospitals, Nicolas Heurteloup, changed Larrey's orders from Toulon to Nice. There Larrey was to establish a surgical staff for the Army of the Maritime Alps. At Nice, he undertook this difficult task, aided by the Jacobin physician from Chambéry, François Doppet, who was now a brigadier general in that army.[20]

The revolt of Lyon was a severe blow to the Convention because the city served as a general supply depot for the military hospitals of four armies: the Alps, Italy, Eastern Pyrenees, and Western Pyrenees. Food and supplies for the ambulance services of these armies also came from Lyon, and the largest and best military hospital outside of Toulon was there.[21]

Further critical weaknesses arose from the Jacobin purging of hospital personnel. There are many good examples in their own reports of how the medical service was hampered by some of these political zealots. For example, the hospital at Embrun was badly needed by the Army of the Alps. Barras and Fréron, after visiting Embrun, told the Committee of Public Safety, "We have discovered a nest of nuns .... All were clothed as in 1788. We have scared the life out of that troop of sisters, who numbered about twelve."[22] Gauthier, with the Army of the Alps, said that food, supplies, and supply wagons were scarce and that many abuses, "tolerated for too long," hampered the proper operation of the military hospitals. He advised that he had planned to attack these problems, but the revolt at Lyon had upset everything.[23]

While General Carteaux, the painter, repulsed an army of rebels from Marseilles, General Doppet retook Avignon on July 27, but no military hospital facilities existed for his casualties. Two Jacobin agents who accompanied Doppet to Avignon, J. S. Rovère and François Poultier, absurdly claimed to have put a new hospital in service at no expense, "as if by magic," and proclaimed it "the most beautiful in the Republic."[24] Since hospitals were among the first buildings damaged around Lyon, casualties from the fighting there had to be taken to Vienne and Valence, while the wounded from the Maritime Alps and Savoy were taken to Avignon and to a hospital set up at Grenoble. Such facilities had been put together only on a temporary basis by ruthless requisitioning without any thought as to how they would continue to operate. By October 10, the need of sustaining support for them was critical. Barras and Fréron pleaded with the Convention: "The hospitals absolutely lack funds: order the Minister of the Interior to send them immediately. This object cannot stand further discussion or delay."[25]

The armies of the Pyrenees were even more desperately in need of medical facilities. No great hospitals existed in the rugged mountain terrain, and evacuation of the wounded posed almost insurmountable problems. In the western Pyrenees, evacuation to Bordeaux from Mont-de-Marsan was impossible. The first roads across the Landes were not cut until the time of Napoleon. A single overland route existed through Tarbes, Mirande, and Auch to Toulouse. At the old Roman city of Dax, where there was one hospital, the representative Michelon had opened an evacuation route through Peyrehorade and Sorde, up the Gave and Adour rivers. The Midouze River could not be used for evacuations except by sled after it froze over, because of the difficulty of navigating it. In addition to the dangers of rapids and of the enemy practice of firing upon boats full of wounded, the evacuees and doctors alike died of dysentery, hospital fever, typhoid fever, and typhus.

In the period 1793–95, Bayonne, Saint Sever, and Dax and their environs were contaminated with the itch, dysentery, and typhus. A high percentage of the wounded contracted tetanus.[26] During an eight-week period in the summer of 1793, every nurse who started work in one typhus-ridden hospital died, as well as three physicians, fourteen surgeons, and eleven apothecaries. General Dugommier, commanding the Army of the Eastern Pyrenees, described his military hospitals as being in "a fearful state," adding that "the most robust health would be ruined in a few days there, and the men constantly tried to get out of them whilst the sick were carted to the rear as so many spoilt goods."[27] The radical Féraud, with the Army of the Western Pyrenees, reported essentially the same conditions to the Committee of Public Safety around July 3, 1793, "It is scandalous," he wrote, "that they have brought our men into hospitals more likely to kill them than to be of any relief to them."[28]

Earlier the zealot Féraud had set up what he called a hospital in the town of Arreau, but he continually complained of "the surgeons, whose ignorance and obstinance are such that they actually have eight hundred patients in the hospital [simply] because of the excessive heat . . . . " On July 3, he announced an incredible accomplishment: the formation of "a general ambulance system covering all points," which was reportedly capable of handling about 5,000 sick and wounded. In addition to making unbelievable claims of his own achievements, Féraud constantly complained about the uncooperative spirit of the local committees of health and demanded that they be investigated by the Committee of Public Safety. The armies of the Pyrenees lacked arms, food, and "generals possessing public confidence," Féraud reported, and he gave the committee a full account of the actions he was taking "to establish order and propriety in the hospitals . . . where the incapacity and the negligence of the health officers are remarkable."[29]

The Jacobin Dagobert, with the Army of the Eastern Pyrenees, observed the battle of Trouillas on September 21, 1793, where the physician Goguet, as brigadier general, was in command of the right wing of the Army of the Eastern Pyrenees. The engagement was bloody but indecisive because Goguet, getting revenge for Dagobert's "sneers" at him, went "skulking off into the woods when he was supposed to turn the Spanish left flank."[30] Desertion was widespread after Trouillas. Dagobert reported to the Committee of Public Safety on September 29 that the patients at the military hospital in Perpignan had not returned to their battalions after discharge. Even worse, some in the battalions were pretending to be sick in order to get hospitalized and then go home.[31]

Military physicians were blamed for desertions from the hospitals, and their relations with the Convention's political agents became increasingly bitter because of the reputations of generals such as Goguet or Doppet. The latter had helped Carteaux retake Marseilles on August 25 and was at Lyon until its surrender on October 9. Doppet was then transferred to Toulon on November 10. Napoleon, who knew him there, declared Doppet to be "an enemy of all talent and so thoroughly a Jacobin as to believe that, when an English shell blew up the magazine battery, it was the work of aristocrats."[32] By November 28, Doppet was transferred to a command in the Army of the Eastern Pyrenees. He spent the next two and one-half months in bed sick and was so ineffective that a reportedly common query of soldiers in the south of France was "When will they

stop sending painters [Carteaux] and doctors [Doppet] to command us? "
Dagobert repeatedly bombarded the Committee of Public Safety with
reports about "these cowardly doctors, improvised generals, whose
shameful inaction has ruined everything."[33]

With active war fronts along the Pyrenees and the Alps as well as in the
North, the need for a unified French military medical service became
increasingly obvious. Various plans had been drafted since 1789 but were
pigeonholed and lost during the hectic years that followed. In the
continuing debate over new national policies on health, welfare, and
education, the subject of a comprehensive health service for the armies had
always been deferred. Even those who urgently wanted an independent
medical service for the armies could not agree upon its proper
organization, although nearly all of the proposals made by medical officers
tended to some extent to follow the familiar pattern of pre-Revolutionary
service.

Of the various plans presented in the spring of 1793, perhaps the most
significant was the one by an ophthalmologist-surgeon, Louis Bernard
Guérin. The title, "Hierarchical Military Surgico-Medical Organization,"
revealed the new status that military surgeons had won on the battlefield
and which they sought to enact into law. Originally drawn up for
presentation to the Legislative Assembly, Guérin's proposal owed much to
abortive earlier plans drawn up by Coste and Percy. Now, in the crisis of
1793, it was Guérin who begged the Convention "to consider the
importance of medical study and practice and to give immediate attention
to the formation of a regular military medical service and abolish the
distinction between physician and surgeon."[34]

His proposal contained concepts important enough to merit a brief
summary and analysis of them. First of all, he proposed that medical
education be hospital-centered and feature practical medicine and surgery,
with the curriculum emphasizing physics, physiology, anatomy, common
illnesses, various surgical techniques, and the treatment of wounds. Only
first- and second-class hospitals would be teaching hospitals; third-class
hospitals would provide medical services only. In the teaching hospitals,
examinations given three times a year would determine who graduated
with the right to practice medicine, surgery, or pharmacy and who would
go to an amphitheatre for further study. The first-class hospitals would
have amphitheatres for top students, and all professors and assistant
professors would be chosen by competitive examinations, with vacancies
to be filled by consultation of students, nominees, and the chief medical
officer. Graduates of the amphitheaters would be attached to cavalry
regiments or demi-brigades. Every hospital would have a hierarchy of

medical men up to chief surgeon, chief pharmacist, and chief consulting physician-surgeon. To supervise the whole structure, a commission of eight physician-surgeons and three pharmacists would act under the rules and supervision of the Committee of Public Welfare. The commission alone, however, would judge the competence of health officers.

In an overall program that does not seem to be too different from the old military medical system, certain key new concepts are visible: first, opportunities for medical training and promotion based upon ability and merit; second, the equality of surgeons with physicians, with a hint that surgeons might come first; third, a rejection of theoretical, systematic medicine for the practical and clinical approach; and fourth, a view of the hospital as the appropriate place for medical care and, rather than universities, for medical education. A comparison with the concepts prevalent only five years earlier will reveal how significantly thinking had changed in the field of medicine. Beliefs which had been held by only a small minority in 1788 had won acceptance among medical men; in 1793 Guérin's proposal did not seem to them to be revolutionary.

Guérin's proposal for a military medical organization was presented to the Committee on Public Welfare because his third-class hospitals were reserve facilities designed to offer public assistance. On March 1, the Convention had already received a proposal from the Council of Health for organizing the military hospital service.[35] It was returned to the Committee of Health to be combined with Guérin's plan and thus to achieve a comprehensive program for a military medical service. Many in the Convention had now become alarmed by the shortage of qualified physicians and surgeons on duty with the armies. Carnot had complained in January of the lack of medical education, as had Fouché in March, and Lakanal in July, but the Convention was being pressured strongly to satisfy a groundswell of demand for free public education. Its Committee of Public Education recognized the need to provide the armies with qualified medical men, even admitted the necessity of reestablishing medical education. But it grimly insisted on settling first the fundamental principles of a revolutionary educational system.[36]

By June 26, 1793, Lakanal was a member of the committee, and he presented a plan for public education that the Convention had published under the title *Projet d'éducation du peuple française*. This proposal envisioned one school for every thousand school-age inhabitants of France. Each *école nationale* would contain two divisions—one for boys and one for girls. The system was designed to give all children some intellectual, moral, and physical education. It would be supported by taxation, with the heaviest burden falling on those who had no children. The proposed law did not provide for any education above the primary level.

Children were to be enrolled at the age of six and both sexes taught together during the first year. They would be separated in the second year. Early subjects were to be arithmetic, reading, and spelling. Later, students would take up geometry, physics, geography, morals, and social studies. Boys would get military training. Advancement was to be on the basis of accomplishment to be measured by regularly administered examinations.

Lakanal's proposal called for a Bureau of Inspection in each school district. The bureau, composed of three members, would be responsible for the quality of administration, the teaching, and the physical plant of each *école nationale*. It would also provide each school with the services of a health officer for the students and teachers. A Central Commission of Instruction was provided for to supervise the district bureaus. The former would set standards on a national scale and see to it that the various bureaus were performing satisfactorily. This Central Commission, composed of twelve members and located in Paris, would be elected annually by the national legislative assembly.[37]

Opposition to Lakanal's plan was vehement. Conflicting theories of education had articulate spokesmen in the Convention, the newspapers, and in the streets. Prudhomme was one of those arguing for no state schools at all, maintaining the ability of the French people to establish a private school system. Bouquier, on the other hand, was among those wanting no formal school system at all, insisting that "The civic, moral, and physical development of French youth could best be met by their attendance at the meetings of representative assemblies and popular societies, by their participation in organized military drills and public festivals, and by apprenticeship in a manual trade."[38]

As the acrimonious debate continued, opposition came from some who felt that Lakanal's scheme was insufficiently equalitarian in its philosophy; others feared that a Central Commission of Public Education would become just another hated academy, and many deputies from the provinces were determined that Paris would not control the new school system. A hatred of any form of "aristocracy" and the prevailing sentiment against academicians continued to frustrate plans for an educational system, and, despite the critical need for medical training, the Convention even refused to utilize the dormant College of Surgery because it was viewed as "a form of aristocracy."[39]

While the great Committee of Public Safety was slowly being formed in the summer of 1793, Lakanal's proposal was subject to further debate. It was evident to most Jacobins that the academies stood in their way and hampered their attempts "to realize moral ideals of justice, equality, and dignity in political institutions."[40] Few educational plans had failed to try to revive the academies under one guise or another. Therefore, on August 8, 1793, a Convention decree abolished all academies and literary societies in France and placed their libraries, equipment, and other assets under governmental supervision. This time, along with the College of Surgery, even the great Academy of Sciences was suppressed. The Committee of Public Safety took over the important medical and scientific projects of these institutions on August 20, although at the same time it vigorously urged the Commitee of Public Education to hurry a report on a reorganized system of education, especially for the desperately needed medical and surgical training.[41]

In the meantime, the Convention received suggestions concerning proposed regulations to govern the admission of candidates to the study of surgery. The implications of inequality in this action immediately provoked a wild and clamorous debate in the Convention. Fourcroy, now a member of the Committee of Public Education, pressed hard for a renewal of medical education, pleading for "physicians and surgeons to comfort suffering men and to ease the bitterness of war . . . ."[42] Anti-intellectuals, such as Coupé de l'Oise, Chabot, and Fabre l'Eglantine, fought Fourcroy's proposal with a savage assault on "sciences and savants." Portiez spoke violently against "Gothic universities" and "aristocratic academies," concluding by blasting Fourcroy with the epithet "academician." Capping the attack of the anti-intellectuals was Bouquier, who informed the Committee of Public Education that: "Free nations have no need of a caste of speculative savants, whose mind wander constantly . . . in the realm of dreams and illusions."[43]

The great chemist Antoine Lavoisier presented his own comprehensive educational plan to the Convention, reflecting in many ways the earlier ideas of Talleyrand, Condorcet, and Mirabeau. The reappearance of such "aristocratic" ideas in August of 1793 only served to heighten the emotional intensity of the fiery controversy over education. Lavoisier's arrest by the Convention on the charge of having been a tax farmer for the Crown added more fuel to the flames of disagreement, and in the late summer of 1793, education in France still lay paralyzed.[44]

It is possible to understand how the bitter debate over the nature of a new educational system for revolutionary France could have been so prolonged. The theoreticians of education were not engaged in a simple political debate where compromise was possible. Rather, as L. Pearce Williams has said, they were locked in a struggle that "involved basic ideological principles concerning the nature of man and of society." Having destroyed the old system, the Jacobins could not agree upon new institutions and new educational practices because "they could not agree upon the theoretical foundations of their new society."[45] This was very evident in the adamant positions around which the debates in the Convention revolved: " . . . the creation of enlightenment and virtue through the study of sciences; the development of public virtues by the indoctrination of youth in the stern values of duty, patriotism, and self-sacrifice; the stimulation of natural virtue by surrounding young men with simplicity and justice so that the inclinations of their hearts could bear fruit in action. No position lacked its ardent defenders but no compromise could be reached."[46]

Since French medical schools had long been considered mere refuges for the unenlightened and the medical profession had been thought a stronghold of privilege and charlatanism, it is not difficult to see why the Jacobins were willing to paralyze the medical schools even at a time when physicians and surgeons were vitally needed during the campaigns of 1792 and 1793. The debate over renewing surgical training "came in the late summer of defeat, alarm, and treason, in the months when the Jacobin regime was establishing its extraordinary efficacy on a rising curve of idealism, patriotism, and terror,"[47] and those who had fought so savagely to destroy the old system were adamantly opposed to restoring any academician to a teaching position. At a time when most physicians were held to be ignorant quacks, when "knowledge came to be considered as a form of aristocracy and genius as a sort of crime against equality,"[48] even a faculty of medicine or of surgery to train badly needed army doctors was repugnant to the aims and ideals of many of the radical Jacobins. Unable to agree upon any new system of education and unwilling to return to the old, most Jacobins were resigned to providing no medical training at all rather than to compromising their educational theories and revolutionary ideals.

Therefore the crisis of 1793 compelled the Committee of Public Safety to assume responsibility for all aspects of French medicine. To help finance the continued operation of hospitals, a subsidy of 8 million livres was announced on July 14, 1793, and another of 10 million livres on February 1, 1794. Physicians, surgeons, and pharmacists were sent on missions to control epidemics and were furnished with money and medical supplies. Following long established practices, the Committee also sent free medicines and money to local physicians to help indigent victims of epidemic illnesses. Where communities had no one to help with medical problems, the Committee drafted physicians and pharmacists from the towns and paid the expenses involved in relocating them.[49]

The Committee took over medical research and the supervision of applied medicine. In June, 1793, Guillaume Daignan was released from the Council of Health to study the nutritive substances of plants which could be useful for convalescents. In August, Corvisart, Hallé, and Portal investigated the use of electricity by one Citizen Sans for healing convulsive seizures in children. They evaluated Sans' methods and reported favorably to the Committee, which then authorized Sans to continue his work. In October the Committee authorized Demours to continue his research on eye diseases, especially the ophthalmia which was raging in the armies. Laumonier, the chief physician at the Humanité in Rouen, was given fifty pounds of mercury from the nation's very short supply in November so that he could continue his research on the lymph glands. By the fall of 1793, the Committee had set up a factory for manufacturing artificial limbs for the amputees who were streaming back from the armies.[50]

The extreme gravity of the war crisis in the late summer of 1793 had finally forced the Great Committee of Public Safety to try to lift the question of medical training out of the morass of debate on educational theory. A proposal to create an independent military medical service, pending in the Convention since March, was enacted on August 7, 1793. This legislation reflected the best thinking of various military officers, including Coste, Percy, Sabatier, Guérin, and others. It embodied many of the new ideas about the proper organization of a medical service which these men had been collecting after the campaign of 1792. The expedient of a close but informal cooperation between line officers and medical men, which had been used in 1792, was abandoned in favor of a more ideal independent medical corps under its own hierarchy of officers.[51]

The Law of August 7 provided for an autonomous medical corps with an administration centered in the War Ministry. A Central Council of Health was created, including Coste, Heurteloup, Parmentier, Daignan, Bayen, and Sabatier, with Biron as secretary. This council, with the approval of the Minister of War, was to appoint and apportion health officers to the armies and to the military hospitals. The council would command the new medical corps, which was designed with ranks corresponding to those of the regular army in terms of pay, rations, forage, and quarters. The Law of August 7, recognizing an urgent need, authorized the resumption of medical training in the military hospitals at Strasbourg, Lille, Toulon, and Metz.[52]

The French experiment with an independent medical corps, however, came at a time of extraordinary crisis. Normal medical instruction was out of the question: the Convention had authorized no funds for it, and the hospitals designated as teaching centers were in danger. Lille was besieged by Coburg's army, Metz and Strasbourg were threatened by the Prussians, and Toulon fell on August 29 to the British. The number of health officers in service, which had been raised to 2,700 during the first three months of 1793 by accepting anyone claiming some medical knowledge, had fallen off sharply by summer. French military reverses on all fronts had produced an alarming rate of desertion among these new health officers, and the loss of experienced, conscientious surgeons to battle injuries was appalling.[53] In the critical summer of 1793, there were simply not the time, the facilities, or the money for organizing the military medical service that the Law of August 7 envisioned.

To relieve the critical shortage of military surgeons and physicians, the Committee of Public Safety had secured a decree from the Convention on August 1 that "all physicians, surgeons, apothecaries, and health officers are at the disposition of the Provisional Executive Council, to be divided among the armies of the Republic according to the needs of the service."[54] The Convention specified, however, that such factors as capacity, patriotism, and training were to be considered in drafting medical men. The War Ministry's orders of August 31, 1793, to all departments, requiring that they compile rosters of "eligible" physicians, surgeons, and apothecaries, were rather unrealistic, since many of the abler physicians and surgeons had volunteered in 1792. The urgent needs of the armies did not allow time for the military medical service to be, as the Convention desired, "composed of the most enlightened and respected men that the nation can furnish."[55]

The Convention's ideal of securing carefully screened men for medical posts proved to be no more possible than the ideal of an independent medical corps had been, considering the magnitude of the crisis France faced. The medical officers selected to test new men being drafted were provided by the Council of Health with packets containing three questions. They were instructed that, "if the candidates cannot answer all three questions in one sitting, then open only one question a day—and successively from sitting to sitting, so that they cannot know the forthcoming questions." The Council was emphatic on this as being the best and legally authorized way "to assure the capacity and degree of competence of citizens who are destined to functions so delicate and important as officers of the military medical service."[56]

This complicated testing process was simply too slow in a time of crisis, so in September the Committee moved decisively to take complete control over military medicine and expedite matters. Desperately needed medical men were simply drafted without reference to their ability and training. The acute shortage of medical corpsmen, assistants, and stretcher-bearers was met by a decree of the Committee of Public Safety which ordered that "men judged less vital to the military service" should be culled out of the battalions.[57] The Committee also announced a purge of the military medical service: "We have not only to serve the armies but still have to purge the military hospitals of some men, whose ignorance or lack of patriotism are equally dangerous."[58]

As France attempted a total mobilization in the late summer of 1793 to save the Republic from invading armies, the fear of conspiracy and treason led to the arrest or execution of generals who lost battles. This fear equated negligence or incompetence with disloyalty.[59] Terror was also applied to the medical service by the Committee of Public Safety. "Army surgeons . . . felt the hand of the new master" in October of 1793.[60]

Still envisioning an independent medical service for the armies, Percy lashed out at "the visitors, examiners, commissioners, inspectors, agents, delegates, deputies of all types, who go round and round, requisitioning, haranguing, exhorting, threatening health officers."[61] Seemingly unaware of the political and military realities of 1793, Percy angrily proclaimed his independence to one of these representatives: "Citizen, I want you to tell the Minister that the Surgeon-in-Chief of the Army of the Rhine is named Percy, a name which the lowest cannot attaint, that he who bears it is above every threat, and that he needs neither the Minister nor his bureaus."[62] To his bitter amazement, Percy was arrested promptly on suspicion of treason. Only the energetic appeals of his friends and the critical need of his fine talents saved Percy from the revolutionary tribunal.

Representatives on mission used their unlimited powers with vigor. Lacoste, with the Army of the North, found grave negligence in all branches of the medical service and authorized a sweeping purge by local Jacobin leaders. Lagresie, surgeon-in-chief of that army, was arrested shortly after Percy.[63] On October 1, the surgeon-in-chief of the military hospital at Cherbourg was suspended. Though the hospital at Huningue, serving the Army of the Rhine, was found to be "in good order," the fathers who served it were expelled for "their religious fanaticism."[64] In Alsace, St. Just whipped medical men into line, putting an end to their hospitalizing troops with what he judged to be "minor" ailments, and requiring that surgeons remain with the troops on the battlefield or be treated as deserters.[65]

On October 5, Laplanche purged the Sisters of Charity from the reserve hospitals in Loir and Cher, though he admitted that "the needs of the hospitals are considerable." The sisters were arrested and imprisoned by Laplanche and forced to burn their habits, though other linens and the mattresses and featherbeds were confiscated and sent to other hospitals. Carrier, who saw treason everywhere, was at Nantes, appealing to the Committee of Public Safety to "recruit in Paris some brave fathers of families, physicians and surgeons who are Jacobins and Cordeliers, to come to Rennes to assume the functions of health officers in the hospitals." He reported having already purged "employees in supply, forage, housing, and registration," and given their places to "very pronounced patriots," but on October 7, he was just preparing to screen employees of the hospitals. There were no good medical men to Carrier: "All of the old health officers smell of aristocracy; the young ones are *muscadins*, royalist minions and federalists, who slipped into their places to avoid taking their delicate and handsome bodies to the frontiers."[66]

While the purge of medical men and medical staffs continued, General André Dufresnoy, chief physician of the Army of the North, on the eve of Wattignies (October 15) announced a conspiracy to furnish contaminated alcohol solutions to his army surgeons. A number of samples, seized by the representative Laurent, were sent to Paris for a quick analysis. Within twenty-four hours, Berthollet and Monge had run chemical tests to prove the purity of the alcohol solution, but their October 15 report to the Committee of Public Safety was challenged by Robespierre until the chemists drank some of it in the Committee's presence.[67] The hapless Dufresnoy, for his erroneous conspiracy report and also for his protest against the arrest of his commissary chief, was demoted by Laurent and assigned to a small hospital at Saint Omer.[68]

Control of the military medical service passed completely into the hands of the Committee of Public Safety in the fall of 1793. Its authority was asserted through a vigorous use of "representatives of the people" who were directly responsible to the Committee. The Central Council of Health, authorized by the Law of August 7, was never fully formed. Coste, who had been named as its chairman, left Paris late in August on a mission to fight a dysentery epidemic in the Army of the Eastern Pyrenees. During the fall of 1793, he was on a similar mission in the department of the Ouest.[69] The Committee of Public Safety also made good use of the Jacobins in the Convention who were medical men. Their zeal, rather than their profession, apparently explains their varied missions. Duhem was assigned to the Army of the Ardennes, Levasseur and Bô to the Army of the North, Cassanyes to the armies of the Pyrenees, and Lacoste to the Rhine and Moselle armies. Baudot served with the armies of the Rhine and of the Eastern Pyrenees. Jard-Panvillier went to the Vendée, Beauvais de Préau was dispatched to Toulon, Siblot to Marly on September 5 to sell the good of emigrés, and Guillemardet was sent to Versailles on October 8 to receive horses requisitioned by the Committee of Public Safety.[70] There is no evidence, however, that their medical training made them any more understanding of medical men in the field than were the laymen who were sent on mission.

The perilous shortage of medical supplies, instruments, and transport was tackled directly by the Committee of Public Safety and its representatives on mission. All linen rags that could be unraveled to make lint for stuffing into wounds were requisitioned by the Committee of Public Safety on September 27. Its decree of October 8 requisitioned blankets, specifying that, "after having been classified by their weight and dimensions, the heaviest [blankets] will be sent to the hospitals."[71] For transport and evacuation of the wounded, the Committee of Public Safety seized horses and wagons, though resistance to these levies was strong even in the loyal departments. Therefore, an acute shortage of transport persisted. The shortage of horses especially frustrated health officers who were concerned with evacuating the wounded from Wattignies. This led to a serious proposal, perhaps inspired by Larrey's idea, "for establishing a mobile hospital for ill horses."[72]

Representatives on mission seized medical supplies wherever and however they could. The chateaux of émigrés and suspects were ransacked for bedding, blankets, linen for bandages, and any medical instruments or equipment. They stripped the former royal mansion at Rambouillet on October 12, selling its furnishing and confiscating eight hundred mattresses and the pillows, linens, and coverings that went with them. At Lâon the same day, Roux reported that he had seized from suspects three hundred mattresses, which he had moved into the military hospital to be used by the wounded who were sleeping on rags. Couthon forced the medical men in Puy-de-Dôme to give up their instruments to the army's health officers. The representatives sent a steady stream of reports to the Committee of Public Safety, outlining the various and urgent needs of military medicine.[73]

Some advice flowed back from Paris. In response to a query from Leclerc, who had asked what to do with the 17-year-olds who had been caught up in the draft of men of ages 18 through 40, the Committee wrote: "Citizens Desault and Manoury have just opened a free course in anatomy and practical medicine at the Hôtel-Dieu. Send them to Paris to take this course."[74] Soon there were questions about the 15-year-olds and 16-year-olds. "Put them in the nearest military hospital for training," the Committee replied. As for the complaints and requests concerning the huge number of venereals in the armies, the Committee declared, "We have no new suggestions. The exigencies of our situation require that they be held in service."[75]

All of this advice was rather irrelevant out in the field, especially in the fall of 1793. On October 18, Roux wrote to the Committee of Public Safety, advising that everyone was being pressed into service to relieve the sufferings of the very great number of wounded from the French victory at Wattignies. The same day, representatives on mission advised that they were drafting men from the army battalions to serve in the hospitals around Arras.[76] Typical of the state to which many hospitals had been reduced were the conditions found by Berthollet at Poissy. There was no kitchen, no pharmacy, no water, no latrines, and no air circulation. One hundred and eighty "filthy patients" were laid side by side on the dirt floor, "unable to defecate except in some pots and [lying] nose to nose with one another."[77]

The representatives on mission cracked down hard on the medical service after Wattignies (October 16–18). The traditional practice of health officers keeping their distance from the battlefield was now classified as "desertion." They were ordered henceforth "to remain with the men in battle instead of withdrawing safely to the rear."[78] Extremely harsh measures were taken to enforce this order. The Committee of Public Safety issued instructions to all representatives on mission declaring, "This conduct is despicable; we charge you to publicize our firm intention to punish it on the spot in the most rigorous way." The "slackness and indifference" of the medical attendants, stretcher-bearers, and wagon drivers in the evacuation of wounded men were also noted by the committee. On pain of six months in prison, these persons were to be instructed to give "instant obedience."[79]

Military physicians and surgeons continued to be accused of being "disgustingly liberal" in giving hospital beds to men who "only wanted to leave their posts and give themselves to a life of idleness." To stop this abuse, the Committee's October 26 order to all military hospitals required health officers to issue a signed ticket to each man on sick leave, stating his illness. If the man was not sick, the health officer whose name was signed to the ticket was to be reported immediately to the Committee of Public Safety.[80] Any soldier presenting a forged certificate was to be treated as a deserter and shot. Two years in irons was decreed for any medical man found guilty of issuing a certificate for a false illness. To curb the desertion and shirking alleged in transferring men from field hospitals to reserve hospitals in the interior, the Committee of Public Safety required a signed statement by a hospital physician or surgeon describing the patient's illness or wound and specifying the particular hospital to which he was being transferred.[81] Armed with these regulations, the representatives on mission moved rapidly in the fall of 1793 to end the lax handling of hospitalization and the opportunities for desertion that it had constantly presented.

The military tribunals established in the armies by representatives on mission, although merciless with deserters, rebels, and émigrés, were nevertheless somewhat lenient with the troops and even with absentees. As Georges Lefebvre has pointed out, between October 28, 1793, and March 6, 1794, the tribunal of the Army of the Rhine judged 660 accused persons, acquitted 282, and handed down only 62 verdicts of capital punishment.[82] As French fortunes of war improved after Wattignies, obedience and discipline were improved in the medical service as much as in the armies. Most of the medical men drafted into the military medical service in the fall of 1793 had Jacobin leanings anyway, and with the tough policies adopted after Wattignies by the Committee of Public Safety, the problem of deserting or absentee health officers was eased. By December, 1793, some 4,000 medical men were on active duty with the armies.[83]

The impact of the Terror upon the military medical service was essentially that of bringing to bear the iron discipline and ruthless measures necessary to provide manpower, supplies, and equipment for an improvised service that had deteriorated badly during the preceding spring. The Law of August 7 had been good legislation, but the exigencies of a desperate war never permitted its implementation. Therefore military medicine was subjected to the central authority of the Committee of Public Safety through its representatives on mission, who exercised an unlimited authority. The horde of other agents, about whom the medical men constantly complained, disappeared by early 1794. Physicians and surgeons learned to look to the all-powerful representatives on mission for their needs. Most French surgeons were like Larrey, who understood the realities of the time and accepted the Jacobin reorganization of the medical service. Their zeal and enthusiasm for getting things accomplished revived in the fall of 1793, but this time it was under a highly centralized system. The decentralized medical service, begun in 1788 as an economy move and continued on an improvised basis, had now come back to the same rigid direction from Paris that it had always known. By December 19, 1793, Toulon had been won back from the British, Lyon had been subdued, the Vendéean rebels routed, and republican armies had halted or thrown back invading armies on every front. In the face of these achievements, there were few who did not accept the policies of the Committee of Public Safety for tightening up and sharply disciplining the military medical service in the same way that the nation had been mobilized and regimented for survival.

NOTES

1. Aulard, *Recueil des actes* 3: 595.

2. Donald Greer, *The Incidence of the Terror During the French Revolution: A Statistical Interpretation* (Cambridge, 1935), pp.31–34.

3. Charles Vellay, "Autographes et documents," *Revue historique de la Révolution française* 12: 175.

4. Nickerson, *Armed Horde*, p.91.

5. Greer, *Incidence of the Terror*, p.34.

6. Guillaume, *Convention* 3: 226.

7. Greer, *Incidence of the Terror*, p.49.

8. Guillaume, *Convention* 1: xc. One of these was the physician Jean Baptiste Salle, finally captured at Bordeaux and executed on June 18, 1794. See Georges Lefebvre, *The French Revolution from 1793 to 1799* (New York, 1964), p.58.

9. Ganges, *Représentants du peuple* 2: 11–12, 270; Vidal, "Cassaynes," *Révolution française* 14: 968.

10. R. R. Palmer, *Twelve Who Ruled* (Princeton, 1941), p.124.

11. Ganges, *Représentants du peuple* 1: 131–32. "The agent of the Council is 'the eye of the Minister' with the armies to discover all treasons, intrigues and abuses. He must give particular attention to visiting the hospitals, and see that our soldiers . . . receive the things to which they are entitled. He must also send a Memoir every month on the materiel of the army, in which he will treat separately hospitals, food, forage, transport, fortifications, artillery, arms, equipment, encampment effects and clothing."

12. Aulard, *Recueil des actes* 5: 231.

13. Ganges, *Représentants du peuple* 2: 268, 403. See Article XVIII.

14. Lefebvre, *French Revolution from 1793 to 1799*, p.48.

15. Aulard, *Recueil des actes* 4: 410.

16. Ibid., 4: 23–43.

17. Percy dossier, carton 211 bis, Val-de-Grâce.

18. Aulard, *Recueil des actes* 4: 34–35.

19. Larrey, *Memoirs* 1: 35–36. On March 4, Larrey was married to Charlotte Leroux, daughter of Louis XVI's finance minister, Laville Leroux. See *Moniteur* 17: 235, and Guillaume, *Convention* 1: 463.

20. Larrey, *Memoirs* 1: 37.

21. Aulard, *Recueil des actes* 4: 245.

22. Ibid., 4: 95.

23. Ibid., 4: 363.

24. Ibid., 6: 266.

25. Ibid., 6: 126, 266; 7: 355.

26. Ferron, "Service de santé," *Arch. de méd. et pharm. mil.* 59: 457, 469.

27. Quoted in Phipps, *Armies of the First Republic* 3: 173

28. Aulard, *Recueil des actes* 5: 162.

29. Ibid., 4: 363, 549; 5: 162, 221.

30. Phipps, *Armies of the First Republic* 3: 158−59.

31. Aulard, *Recueil des actes* 7: 127.

32. Ganges, *Représentants du peuple* 2: 269.

33. Phipps, *Armies of the First Republic* 3: 116, 159.

34. "Organisation chirurgico-médicale hierarchique militaire proposée par le Citoyen Louis Bernard Guérin, le 21 floreal an II," Conseil de Santé documents, carton 12, Arch. hist. Service de Santé.

35. "Projet de décret portant organisation du Service des Hôpitaux militaires presenté à la Convention par les membres du Conseil de Santé, 1 mars 1793," Rapports aux inspecteurs-généraux, carton 21, ibid.

36. *Arch. parl.* 58: 17; 59: 710; 68: 212.

37. Joseph Lakanal, *Projet d'éducation du peuple française* (Paris, 1793), pp.6−8.

38. John R. Vignery, *The French Revolution and the Schools: Educational Policies of the Mountain, 1792−1794* (Madison, 1965), pp.128, 230−31.

39. Guillaume, *Convention* 4: xxxii; Fayet, *La Révolution et la science*, p.471.

40. From Charles Coulston Gillispie, "The *Encyclopédie* and the Jacobin Philosophy of Science: A Study in the Ideas and Consequences," in Marshall Clagett, ed., *Critical Problems in the History of Science* (Madison, 1959), p.256. Gillispie insists that "once affairs were engrossed by Jacobinism, science was bound to incur the enmity of the Republic. This is not because scientists were unpatriotic. On the contrary, they pressed into the service of the State on a scale unequalled until the twentieth century. But in its intrinsic combination of assurance and irrelevance, science all unintentionally stood across the cosmic ideals of the Republic in a posture nonetheless insulting for being unassumed."

41. *Arch. parl.* 70: 519−24; 72: 472. The *Moniteur* of August 8 treated this action lightly, giving only a few lines to it. Gillispie, "The *Encyclopédie* and the Jacobin Philosophy of Science," *Critical Problems*, p.257, says that friends of the Academy of Sciences on the Committee of Public Education inserted five clauses in an effort to give provisional

continuation to the Academy of Sciences, but a single speech by David forced their withdrawal. Both Guillaume and Fayet agree that Grégoire ⁻lied in his memoirs when he claimed that his proposed decree of August 8 intended to exempt from abolition the Academy of Sciences, the College of Surgery, the Society of Medicine, and the Society of Agriculture. See Guillaume, *Convention* 2: 246—47, and Fayet, *La Révolution et la science*, p.122.

42. Fayet says that the hatred of savants reflected a demand for a complete break with the past. Insisting that "knowledge came to be considered as a form of aristocracy and genius a sort of crime against equality," Fayet concludes that this explains why many Frenchmen were willing to paralyze their medical schools even when they desperately needed physicians and surgeons. Ibid., p.209. See also Guillaume, *Convention* 2: 85.

43. Guillaume, *Convention* 3: 56. "The Republic has no need of savants" has been a phrase much debated by historians of the Terror. Albert Mathiez, "Mobilisation des savants en l'an II" *Revue de Paris* 24: 549, noted its attribution by historians to both Coffinhal and to Dumas but said that the statement was probably never uttered. Guillaume, "Un mot légendaire," *Révolution française* 38: 385, calls the statement "a Thermidorean legend" and "apocryphal." Pouchet, "Les sciences pendant la terreur," ibid., 30: 347, attributes the statement to Fourcroy but admits that it is probably an apocryphal saying. On the other hand, Fayet, *La Révolution et la science*, p.197, is convinced that Coffinhal probably did make the statement. The remark made by Bouquier, quoted above, closely approximates this phrase and may have been its source. In any event, Bouquier's statement is not apocryphal and it clearly expresses the strong anti-intellectualism that Pouchet doubts, that Guillaume rejected as "legend," and that Mathiez denied.

44. Edouard Grimaux, *Lavoisier, 1743—1794, d'apres sa correspondance, ses manuscrits, ses papiers de famille et d'autre documents inédits* (Paris, 1896), p.243, depicted Fourcroy as a ruthless enemy of the Academy of Sciences and of Lavoisier. He charged that Fourcroy alone was responsible for Lavoisier's fate (p.200), insisting that he made no effort to save Lavoisier (p.278). The accusations by Grimaux have been thoroughly discredited by Pouchet, "Les sciences pendant la terreur," *Révolution française* 30: 255, 347; by McKie, *Lavoisier*, pp.338—42; by Smeaton, *Fourcroy*, pp.42—43; 46—49, 56; and by Guillaume, *Convention* 3: 56; 4: 379.

45. From L. Pearce Williams, "The Politics of Science in the French Revolution," in Clagett, *Critical Problems in the History of Science*, p.304.

46. Ibid., p.301.

47. From Gillispie, "The *Encyclopédie* and the Jacobin Philosophy of Science," *Critical Problems*, p.257.

48. Fayet, *La Révolution et la science*, pp.209, 471.

49. *Arch. parl.* 56: 644; Aulard, *Recueil des actes* 12: 753; 18: 544; 20: 542; Guillaume, *Convention* 4: 58.

50. Conseil de Santé documents, carton 13, Arch. hist. Service de Santé; Rapports aux inspecteurs-généraux, carton 21, ibid.

51. Rapports aux inspecteurs-généraux, carton 21, ibid.

52. Ibid. See also Cilleuls, "Les médecins aux armées," *Revue hist. de l'armée* 6: 16 and Garrison, *Notes*, p.162. The simplicity and practicality of this legislation served as a model for reforms being made at the same time in England by John Hunter. Appointed Surgeon-General of the Army in 1793, Hunter's first move was to destroy the old system that had permitted the medical colleges to monopolize army medical appointments. Before his death on October 16, John Hunter had given England an independent medical corps wherein commissions were bestowed upon meritorious physicians and surgeons equally after specified terms of service in the ranks. See Kobler, *John Hunter*, pp.295, 305.

53. Rieux and Hassenforder, *Histoire*, p.20; Cilleuls, "Les médecins aux armées," *Revue hist. de l'armée*, 6: 24.

54. Augustin Cochin and Charles Charpentier, eds., *Les actes du gouvernement Révolutionnaire (23 aôut 1793–27 juillet 1794). Recueil de documents publiés pour la Société d'histoire contemporaine* (Paris, 1920–35), 1: 19–20; Laws and Decrees, carton 1, Arch. hist. Service de Santé; Aulard, *Recueil des actes* 18: 71.

55. Rapports aux inspecteurs-généraux, carton 21, Arch. hist. Service de Santé; Cochin and Charpentier, *Les actes* 1: 19–20.

56. Rapports aux inspecteurs-généraux, carton 21, Arch. hist. Service de Santé.

57. Aulard, *Recueil des actes* 17: 620–21.

58. Cochin and Charpentier, *Les actes* 1: 19–20.

59. Lefebvre, *French Revolution from 1793 to 1799*, pp.96–97; Mathiez, "Mobilisation des savants," *Revue de Paris* 24: 549.

60. Palmer, *Twelve Who Ruled*, p.183.

61. Laurent, *Percy*, p.153. Also see the account of this in Triaire, "Tactique sanitaire," *Caducée* 2: 158.

62. Percy dossier, carton 211 bis, Val-de-Grâce; Laurent, *Percy*, pp.158–60, 188.

63. Aulard, *Recueil des actes* 7: 278–88; Laurent, *Percy*, p.188.

64. *Arch. parl.* 49: 289; Aulard, *Recueil des actes* 19: 187.

65. Palmer, *Twelve Who Ruled*, p.183.

66. Aulard, *Recueil des actes* 7: 236–37; 287.

67. Dufresnoy dossier, carton 206/1, Val-de-Grâce.

68. Armées du Nord, carton 25, Arch. hist. Service de Santé. At St. Omer, Dufresnoy was later arrested because his intercepted letter to a physician in Cambrai requested some rhus plants. This was offered as evidence that Dufresnoy had been corresponding with the Russians. He

was saved from execution by the events of 9 Thermidor.

69. Coste dossier, carton 205/1, Val-de-Grâce.

70. Aulard, *Recueil des actes* 5: 56; 6: 285; 7: 301; Guillaume, *Convention* 2: xcii; Ganges, *Représentants du peuple* 1: 346; 2: 12, 202.

71. Aulard, *Recueil des actes* 7: 297; Mathiez, "Mobilisation générale en l'an II," *Revue de Paris* 24: 595.

72. Conseil de Santé documents, cartons 11 and 12, Arch. hist. Service de Santé; Aulard, *Recueil des actes* 7: 301, 311, 380–82, 478.

73. Aulard, *Recueil des actes* 6: 383; 7: 233, 574; Palmer, *Twelve Who Ruled*, p.140.

74. Rapports aux inspecteurs-généraux, carton 21, Arch. hist. Service de Santé.

75. Conseil de Santé documents and correspondence, carton 20, ibid.; Rapports aux inspecteurs-généraux, carton 21, ibid.

76. Aulard, *Recueil des actes* 7: 484, 487.

77. Cabanès, *Médecins amateurs*, p.339. Reproduction of the original of a report by Berthollet to the Committee of Public Safety which was in Cabanès's private collection.

78. Palmer, *Twelve Who Ruled*, p.183.

79. Ganges, *Représentants du peuple* 1: 329.

80. Cochin and Charpentier, *Les actes* 1: 312–13.

81. Ibid., 3: 269; Aulard, *Recueil des actes* 17: 628.

82. Lefebvre, *French Revolution from 1793 to 1799*, pp.97–98.

83. Coste dossier, carton 205/1, Val-de-Grâce. See folio A.

Chapter Seven

BATTLE SURGERY

Many of the great battle surgeons who followed Napoleon to Italy, Egypt, Spain, and Russia first learned to cope with the horrible mutilations of war as neophytes in the armies of the First Republic. Confronted with injuries of a magnitude and variety unimagined in peacetime, these surgeons, hampered by a lack of equipment and supplies, experimented and improvised means of caring for overwhelming numbers of casualties. The good ones acquired what Briot termed "a noble audacity."[1] Percy described their approach in a similar vein: "The art of healing men is a little like that of destroying them; timidity gains nothing and, if victory often follows the audacity of brave soldiers, success also crowns the efforts of enterprising surgeons."[2]

The Revolution had given military surgeons an equal standing with physicians, but the war years after 1792 saw them gain an actual ascendancy over physicians. There were several reasons for this change. Physicians carried with them into military service the secret potions and complicated treatments upon which their civilian reputations were based, while wartime conditions afforded only a few simple medicinals that were easy to supply and administer. Still clinging to their speculative schools of medical thought, physicians brought to the ailments of the armies only the traditional theories of disease and the conventional modes of civilian practice. When faced with wartime epidemic illnesses, the virtual helplessness of practitioners of the "old medicine" was painfully obvious. Surgeons, on the other hand, approached the sick and wounded with fewer preconceived notions and simpler tools. On the field of battle the one who could help the wounded best was the surgeon; and under conditions that were hazardous and unfamiliar, he proved best able to adapt, to improvise, and to experiment. Officers and troops alike quickly evidenced their faith in and preference for the military surgeon.

The problem of battle wounds was one of great complexity even for well-trained surgeons. Punctures by bayonets and sabres differed from those made by smooth-bore rifle balls. Shell fragments produced torn, jagged wounds; sabres delivered sharp, deep gashes. Injuries inflicted by bayonets and sabres were usually clean, but gunshot wounds were almost always complicated by the presence of clothing fragments or other foreign particles.[3] Unlike the hardened bullets of a later time, the soft lead balls of the eighteenth century flattened on impact and shattered bones. In addition to the shock that accompanied many wounds, burns and concussions from exploding shells, cannon, or powder magazines complicated the surgeon's task. Briot learned that there were so many reactions to so many different wounds and so many factors involved in treating a wound that even similar wounds had to be handled differently "according to whether [they are] received at the beginning . . . or at the end of a battle."[4]

Bullet punctures of the fleshy parts usually produced so little immediate pain that many men did not know they had been wounded until the battle was over. The surgeons had to learn to estimate that nearly half of all wounds were made by bullets in the soft parts of the body. This factor was important to take into account in preparation and arrangement of dressings. The old smooth-bore bullets generally inflicted a contusion and remained in the "cul-de-sac" wound, rather than making a through-and-through perforation. Some who were hit immediately dug the ball out of their flesh by themselves. From many accounts of this, the case of Pierre Lafargue, a volunteer of the 2nd Battalion of Lot-et-Garonne, may be cited. Wounded in the Rhinefeld woods late in 1792 by a bullet in his hip, he "had the courage to dig it out himself, load it in his gun and return it to the enemy, saying: 'Look, here is how republicans fight'."[5] Briot captured the nonchalance of the walking wounded who came back to his mobile hospital for aid: "Here comes a soldier with a gunshot wound; the ball appears to be accessible to our extracting instruments, the man is placed at once in the most convenient position; two incisions, if they are deemed necessary, quickly lay open the area and facilitate the search, and then one does not know who is the most pleased, the surgeon who presents the ball to the patient or the patient who receives it from the surgeon's hand."[6]

At other times, wounded men exhibited immediate and violent reactions, such as convulsions or vomiting. Some superficial wounds appeared to be massive; other wounds appeared to be slight but the internal havoc was enormous. Artillery shells splintered bones and tore flesh savagely; the victims most gravely injured only moaned or lay mute in shock while those less dangerously hurt filled the air with their screams of agony.[7]

Given such a gamut of wounds and reactions to wounds, the French military surgeon of the 1790s had to practice surgery in much the same way that French generals were making war. It was a matter of knowing what resources he had on hand and, expecting no supplies or reinforcements, making the necessary use of them for the greatest degree of success. Often lacking the most indispensable items, the military surgeon learned on the battlefield how to adapt what he had to the needs of his wounded men. A pocket scalpel often served to make every sort of incision and nearly every type of operation. A simple probe (or his fingers if necessary) helped to locate and extract balls, bone splinters, and pieces of clothing. Simple tweezers were utilized instead of whatever instrument the specific case required. The thumb pressed on a vein supplying a hemorrhage served to stop it until a thread could tie it off. Simple bandages, designed by necessity, often served several purposes at once, such as compensating for a lack of sutures or for the absence of compresses.[8]

In the revolutionary armies, the battlefield surgeon was usually as ill-equipped as the troops. The only really plentiful commodity for bathing wounds was water, and often it was the entire medication for even the most serious injuries. Any available rag provided the lint to moisten and stuff into wounds but, lacking that, leaves, grass, and moss did just as well. Lacking ordinary meat with which to make soup for their wounded, surgeons found horsemeat a good substitute, and in the absence of salt, the soup could be seasoned with gunpowder. Improvisation and ingenuity were the principal assets of the military surgeon who, in the midst of scores of wounded, had to judge who could be saved, who needed him most, and what kind of help he could give.[9]

Many of the surgeons who enlisted in 1792 and 1793 had much to learn but much to forget as well. Perhaps the most universal practice of the time was that of inserting a drain (*seton*) into a wound made by a rifle ball. Writing in 1817, Briot observed: "So great a number of old surgeons were enslaved to that false practice that, to my astonishment, I find it still advised in an elementary work on surgery which is otherwise worthy to be a textbook for students." He and Percy, "who believed in the resources of nature in wound healing," fought constantly against the traditional use of the *seton*.[10] An equally common procedure was the use of the fingers to probe into wounds. Many surgeons, oblivious to the consequences, continued this quite murderous practice despite the efforts of the top military surgeons to stop it. Briot, who said that in the period 1792–98 he "never used or saw used" the fancy bullet-extractors of Thomassin (*curette-tire-balle*) or of Percy (*tribulcon*), favored using a simple dressing forceps.[11]

Almost every surgical student knew that the continued presence of a foreign object in a wound hindered its healing. Many, like Briot, believed that "its presence changes the normal rhythm of the vital forces of the tissues with which it is in contact," thus producing complications. The urge to probe a wound and attempt to remove a bullet or a bone fragment was therefore almost irresistible to young surgeons. They had had opportunities to observe not only the complications caused by foreign objects left in a wound but, according to Briot, they learned that these foreign objects tended to move around, and though originally located in a harmless spot, could in time move to a vital spot. Even balls, which were ordinarily smooth and round, if left embedded soon developed points or ragged, sharp edges capable of doing great internal mischief. All surgeons knew the good effect that extraction had upon the morale of the wounded man, and they generally held to the conviction that "one ought to try to operate while the foreign body was accessible and before it compressed a nerve or a lymph vessel or a blood vessel, occasioned paralysis, interrupted circulation, occasioned swelling in nearby parts, produced listlessness, convulsions, [or] tetanus . . . . "[12]

Such compelling reasons for probing wounds were reinforced by the time-honored precept that surgeons should make one or two incisions in a wound. This not only aided the removal of any foreign object; also, as Briot observed, the practice of wound excision was "a residue of that idea held in the past that the wound was poisoned, and that it was necessary to bleed wounds promptly and to change their shape . . . . "[13] In areas where wound excision was obviously dangerous, such as the brain, the chest, and the abdomen, many military surgeons still pursued their efforts to expel foreign bodies. Men bearing these wounds were required to expectorate, to cough, or were given laxatives, or emetics to induce vomiting. Only much experience in observing the results (hemorrhaging, convulsions, even death) finally persuaded many surgeons to stop these measures. One of them was Briot, who said candidly, "I admit that if I sometimes have conformed to these precepts, I often found myself making a mistake."[14] Because wound excision was so commonly practiced, the best that top military surgeons could do was to try to educate their subordinates as to which wounds were to be left alone because of the danger to the life of the patient.[15]

The shortage of medicines that developed in 1793 also helped to transform the treatment of wounds by military surgeons. Some attempted to continue using messy oils, ointments, plasters, and various solutions for bathing wounds, but supplies of these remedies, usually invented and prepared by individual surgeons, were almost exhausted after the campaign of 1792. Percy fought strenuously against their use and against the usual practice of stuffing lint soaked in brandy or irritating salves into open wounds, finally issuing an order in 1793 forbidding it in the Army of the North. Lorentz issued a similar order in early 1794 in the Army of the Rhine.[16]

Larrey's revival of the use of moxa in 1792 was a significant improvement in the treatment of wounds.[17] The hot cautery iron too often produced complications or was used in a manner that did extensive and permanent damage to the patient. The moxa, consisting of a cone or cylinder of combustible materials, could be applied to a wound and then ignited, but the burn it made could be controlled. Light, moderate, or deep burns could be inflicted with a moxa, depending upon the combustibility of the materials used and whether it was perforated to secure slow or fast combustion. In emergencies, dried leaves, moss, or plant stalks could be used, although Larrey recommended linen treated with potassium nitrate or lint treated with acetate of lead.[18] He insisted that it was better to use several light moxas than to burn deeply with one. Larrey also demonstrated the superiority of moxa in treating skin ulcers and in healing abscesses that would have been dangerous to open surgically.[19] Although he had only revived a very old practice, Larrey popularized the use of moxa as an alternative to the cautery iron, and contributed importantly to a better concept of wound treatment.[20]

For bathing wounds, water soon became almost the only commodity available to military surgeons; it was certainly Percy's favorite. He demonstrated the value of water over the old perfumed washes on some sixty volunteers of the Louvre Battalion who had received foot wounds in an attack on Montagne-Verte near Treves on Christmas Day, 1792. By bathing their feet continuously in lukewarm water, Percy healed them promptly.[21] However, the credit for originating wound irrigation should go to Larrey. In an effort to avoid unnecessary amputations, he devised a method of letting a constant stream of water flow on a wound to remove inflammation and help rebuild tissues.[22] Water came to be generally used after 1792, first of necessity and later by choice. Cold water became the standard item for bathing wounds made by sabres, bayonets, swords, and in cases of shock and stupor, while gunshot wounds were treated with lukewarm water if possible. Briot later asserted that military surgeons believed as much or more in the efficacy of water than in all the other remedies combined, and swore: "I will abandon surgery if they forbid me water, just as Suydenham used to say that he would renounce medicine if they deprived him of the use of opium."[23]

Under the wartime necessity of being sparing with their limited medical supplies, surgeons soon reduced the dressing for simple wounds made by rifle balls to a bit of soft wadding dipped in lukewarm water and covered by a compress. In some cases a simple emollient patch, which could be changed as often as needed, could serve the purpose. Where it was necessary to absorb purulent matter, the standard dressing was a plain dry bandage. Most of the surgeons who volunteered in 1792 saw "agglutinative" bandages for the first time. When they were available, these new adhesive bandages were useful for most wounds and even for ulcers.[24]

Briot declared that the bandage was the one thing with which "surgeons of every grade were the most familiar; and it is, I believe, the one that they have most perfected." Testifying to the unexcelled ability of French military surgeons to improvise with bandages, Briot proudly recorded an example of his own ingenuity, made necessary one day when he ran out of sutures: "When I was attached to the flying ambulance near Mayence, they brought me to a soldier who, in a cavalry charge, sustained three sabre cuts on his head . . . . These wounds, the least of which was two thumbs long, ran in different directions. I prepared a long bandage, plus six pieces of linen four thumbs long by two or three thumbs wide: I made holes in some and tongues in others. In succession, I placed each of these linen pieces thus prepared in a direction opposite to those of the wounds. I secured them by several turns of the long bandage; I passed the tongues through the holes, tightened one against the other in an inverse sense, and secured the loose ends with the bandage."[25]

In learning to deal with fractures and dislocations, French military surgeons on the northern front were fortunate to be in the vicinity of the famous amateur country physicians of the Vosges Mountains, called "rebouteurs" or "renoueurs" of Valdajol (Val-d'Ajol). They were not farmers primarily but specialists in osteology, serving their neighbors in a mountainous area where bone fractures and dislocations were common. One of the surgeons who learned from the Valdajols wrote: "They knew how to diagnose and, more than once when encamped with my regiment in the vicinity, I profited from their experience . . . ."[26]

Rebouteurs such as Fleurot and Dumont de Valdajol, taught from childhood by their fathers the mechanics of the skeleton, handled dislocations and fractures with an ease that amazed the military surgeons who watched them. Especially simple to adopt was the rebouteur technique of plying a victim with warm wine until a drunken stupor ensued and allowed the necessary muscular relaxation for the easy setting of a fracture or dislocation. Surgeons who were familiar with Hugues Ravaton's "tin boot" contraption for hip dislocations and leg fractures promptly discarded it as the rebouteur technique became common practice.[27]

Setting broken hips and pelvic bones had always been painful and difficult. This encouraged frequent eighteenth-century clinical experiments with a distillate of tobacco. Injected into the intestines, it was quickly resorbed and produced muscular relaxation. However, fatal nicotine poisonings had resulted in most cases because the effect of the nicotine could not be controlled. A simpler procedure, known to the rebouteurs of the Vosges, was to introduce a strong cigar into the rectum. Resorption took a bit longer, but the cigar could be withdrawn as soon as the proper muscular relaxation occurred.[28] Learning how to relax the great muscles of the abdomen and legs was considered a great breakthrough by the military surgeons who were confronted by so many terrible fractures. Many of the future great surgeons of the Empire, such as Larrey, Percy, Saucerotte, and the great veterinary surgeon of the Empire, Lafosse, learned from the Valdajols and readily acknowledged their debt to them. Larrey was impressed so much by the anesthetic aspects of the rebouteur techniques that he constantly experimented with ways to dull the pain of amputations, most notably anticipating a modern technique by trying refrigeration.[29]

Many field surgeons, equally anxious to mitigate the terrible pain of operations without anesthesia, operated first upon men who seemed to be in a stupor. Simon Boy, surgeon-in-chief of the Army of the Rhine, declared that he had seen wounded men operated upon who were numbed by the cold and observed that they promptly died.[30] Operations upon men in shock almost always produced fatal results but most surgeons, hard-pressed by many casualties, rarely paused to consider shock or stupor. Briot confessed that he made this error many times himself.[31] Only very slowly did French army surgeons learn that shock demanded treatment before any surgery could succeed. The treatment itself was often haphazard, ranging from the use of aromatic spirits, sips of warm sugared wine, and the application of ice, snow, or cold water to "stimulating enemas."[32]

The shock associated with many of the terrible burns that surgeons encountered did not respond well to these treatments, however. Even the traditional treatments for burns, such as applications of cold ammoniated water, opium water, or vinegar water, were found to be injurious. Surgeons gradually came to the view that the massive burns and deep shock produced by gunpowder blasts were treated best when the victim was least disturbed. Larrey taught his surgeons simply to flow a cerate of oil upon the burned area, or if oil were not available, honey. To avoid irritation, fine linen, worn soft, was used to dress the burn. Customarily, Larrey left the dressings on as long as possible to avoid disturbing the patient.[33] This new approach to treating the great searing burns of warfare was a blessing to friend and foe alike. In the Pyrenees, at the Battle of Black Mountain, November 17–18, 1794, the Spanish surrendered after their powder magazine blew up. Amidst the scores of dead, French surgeons found sixty Spaniards, in shock and terribly burned, and saved them all.[34]

Skin grafts for burns were unknown, but Briot successfully experimented with reapplying skin fragments sliced off by sabres. He recalled how, at Mayence on January 2, 1794, he treated a soldier who had been sabred in the head. A portion of the left parietal hump, as well as the tissue fastening the occipito-frontal muscle to the skull, had been cut out and left hanging by only a few matted hairs. After cleaning the wound and the skin fragment, Briot carefully fitted the cut-out flesh back in place. "I found," he said, "that the hairs of the fragment, which I twisted several times to mat with other hairs, seemed to be the best means of fastening the fragment back in place."[35] Several years later, Briot learned indirectly that his operation had been successful.

A fortunate by-product of the lack of surgical instruments by French battle surgeons was an improvement in the treatment of head wounds and skull fractures. The precept of trepanning (relieving pressures by cutting holes in the skull), hallowed by the Academy of Surgery, had become an abuse practiced by countless surgeons. Desault at Paris and Lombard at Strasbourg, however, had taught their students to shun indiscriminate trepanning, and when wartime conditions made it difficult, trepanning was rarely resorted to. Briot, for example, observed that he had seen skull fractures by the hundreds and learned that they healed better and were attended by fewer complications if trepanning was avoided. Often deaths attributed to untreated skull fractures proved to be nothing of the sort. Lombard recalled seven cases at the Strasbourg hospital during January and February of 1794 wherein the patients apparently died of skull fractures, but six of the deaths were found after autopsies to have been due to abcesses of the liver.[36] Therefore, except for those rare cases where trepanning was clearly indicated, surgeons came to be sparing in its use because their experience proved that most patients did better without it.

A better understanding of wounds resulted from the solution of an old battlefield mystery: bodies found on the battlefield without any visible wound. For centuries the cause of these unmarked dead had been attributed to "the wind of the ball" by physicians who thought that the air stirred up by a passing bullet was strong enough to suppress respiration completely. Cases diagnosed in 1792 as "wind deaths" were carefully examined and, in the autopsies performed by Larrey, his students were shown the internal damage done even though no external damage was visible.[37] The explanation that blows on the head, chest, or abdomen, that left no apparent contusion were violent enough to cause death contributed greatly to a new attitude among military surgeons. Old explanations became suspect; more natural explanations for common medical phenomena were eagerly entertained.

The old and poorly understood problem of hemorrhaging gradually yielded to experience derived from new conditions. The lack of hemorrhage in some gunshot wounds and the massive blood flow in others had led to an explanation that differences in age or physical condition of the victims were responsible. The standard teaching on chest wounds with some associated bleeding was excision to facilitate more bleeding until the blood flow coagulated. This traditional practice proved on the battlefield what a few brave spirits had dared to suggest: far from stopping hemorrhage, it in fact maintained it. Briot said that "posterity can very justly attribute to Larrey the honor of having indicated the correct treatment of hemorrhaging chest wounds, just as it credits Harvey with discovery of blood circulation."[38] The practice that evolved in the period 1792–95 was one that many surgeons must have stumbled upon, despite Briot's desire to give credit to Larrey. Briot himself recorded how he found a soldier shot between the fifth and sixth ribs and, sure that the man was dying, merely closed his wound with an agglutinative patch and a body bandage. According to his recollection, Briot learned something about chest wounds from this encounter: "I calculated that his bleeding in the chest would not increase his danger and shortly after the wound was closed the patient breathed more freely and seemed relieved. His color began to return. His pulse grew stronger. He became completely calm and, to my great surprise, the sick man got better and better and [the wound] healed in a few days with no difficulty."[39]

Hemorrhaging in other parts of the body did not respond nearly as well to this simple treatment. The centuries-old practice of cauterizing gunshot wounds with boiling oil had gradually ended under the influence of Ambroise Paré (1510–90). The cautery iron became standard, but eighteenth-century teachers such as Jean Louis Petit had given prominence to the use of compression in cases of severe hemorrhage.[40] An equally prevalent approach to great amputation hemorrhages was to wrap the stump with a bladder containing a small amount of coagulating blood. This latter technique of clinical surgery proved unsuited to battle conditions.

Compression was also rejected by the military surgeons of the 1790s on two grounds. First, experience rapidly told them that compression sufficient to stop a massive hemorrhage ordinarily produced fatal complications, especially in the case of men in shock. Second, they observed that the forced movement or transport of wounded men usually meant that "the compresses were going to get out of place, and they did not want their lives depending upon so fragile and precarious a contrivance."[41]

With hundreds of badly hemorrhaging casualties upon whom they could experiment, French battle surgeons adopted an approach that emphasized speed and practicality. Even with severe hemorrhaging in a limb, the tourniquet was seldom used. The hemorrhage could be stopped more quickly by applying a thumb to the opening in the vein. This easy practice became habitual. With the fingers, an open vein could be pulled up and tied off. Only when there was a great vein buried deep in tissues and difficult to get a ligature around did battle surgeons resort to moxa or to the cautery iron. Both Larrey and Percy taught the ligature of veins and avoided using the iron if at all possible, although most surgeons on the battlefield had to deal with massive hemorrhages in the most practical and immediate fashion.[42]

Some of the most terrible wounds that battle surgeons faced were abdominal. The temptation to remove a ball from the abdomen was virtually irresistible but the result was usually fatal. Despite the efforts of Larrey, Percy, and others to educate their subordinates, the practice continued. General Marceau was lost this way. The surgeon who attended him at Altenkirchen on September 19, 1796, quickly extracted the ball from Marceau's abdomen. Marceau died on September 21, almost predictably, of peritonitis.[43] Briot described the case of a soldier brought to the field hospital at Plaisance in 1793 suffering from a great wound in the abdomen. The battle surgeon who attended the victim had extracted the ball, stuffed the wound with a bit of linen, and covered it with a large emollient bandage. At the hospital, the soldier was immediately bled and then slated for rest and a strict diet. By the fifth day, Briot observed: "The wound became very tender; swelling and inflammation separated its edges and soon revealed nearly everything beneath the abdominal wall. The application of flannel soaked in an emollient solution could scarcely be tolerated. Constipation became chronic and, despite four copious bleedings, the attachment of twenty leeches to the abdomen, lukewarm baths, washing the wound with water, his condition worsened and the patient died on the tenth day."[44]

Such observations as these gradually led to the conclusion that men with abdominal wounds were better off left alone. The complicated laparotomies that were being performed on the battlefield in 1792 and 1793 were always fatal. The practice was condemned and generally abandoned after statistical evidence proved that even men left on the battlefield without food did better than those upon whom laparotomies were attempted.[45] Out of this new respect for abdominal wounds came a safe and easy procedure for dealing with punctures of the bladder, whether by ball or by sabre. Larrey practiced and taught his students catheterization. A catheter inserted into the bladder did not allow it to fill and thus permitted the wound edges to join and heal naturally.[46] Many abdominal wounds, however, were great holes torn by artillery fragments. Battle surgeons could do little for these usually fatal wounds. Still, a few men owed their lives to Sabatier, who taught surgeons how to suture a divided intestine over a cylinder made of an ordinary playing card smeared with turpentine.[47]

Two dread enemies that baffled French military surgeons claimed the lives of thousands and provoked a bitter and sustained controversy over amputation. They were gangrene and tetanus. In 1792, gangrene was commonly pursued by the surgeon's scalpel. Small incisions and then large incisions to secure free drainage, a careful cutting away of infected tissue, and cleaning the wound with water were standard measures aimed at controlling the spread of gangrene. It was known that gangrene was most common in wounds of the thigh, the leg, and the forearm. Larrey and Briot also observed that its worst ravages occurred in hot humid weather and in individuals who "abounded in fatty cell tissue."[48] Larrey soon rejected the prevalent notion that gangrene could be absorbed by the body, and taught that prompt amputation was the sole means of saving the patient.[49] After an unhappy experience with gangrene at Plaisance in December, 1792, Briot came to the same conclusion. His patient was a soldier who had walked four kilometers to the hospital with a sabre cut on the outside of his right knee. Briot applied a pressure bandage to the now badly separated wound, applied poultices, exercised the knee, and bled the patient. He pursued the gangrene with his scalpel into the knee joint, but while allowing free drainage this surgery did not stop the formation of enormous abscesses. Nothing that Briot did relieved the terrible pain nor stopped the spread of gangrene and the soldier soon died. Belatedly, Briot thought that an amputation might have saved his patient.[50]

Tetanus was almost always fatal and, before 1793, it was thought that amputation was not effective in combatting it. Briot was the first to distinguish between what he called "chronic" tetanus, a form that responded to treatment, and "acute" tetanus, which was fatal in a few days.[51] The cause of tetanus remained a mystery. Percy, in 1793, noted that the greatest incidence of tetanus was in hospitals near cannon batteries but drew no conclusion from this fact.[52] The popular explanation was that tetanus arose from violent passions. Jean Jacques Canin noted a patient responding well to opium treatments but who worsened and died suddenly when someone stole his money. Claude Leclerc insisted that he saw greatly frightened men die of tetanus. Another surgeon explained that anger introduced tetanus into the muscular system, while many others confused tetanus with apoplexy and epilepsy.[53]

The treatments for tetanus were as widely varied as the explanations. Auenbrugger had taught the use of mercury. Newer eighteenth-century discoveries, electricity and castor oil, were tried by others. In 1793, Lorentz and Lombard were using purgatives while Larrey prescribed opium mixed with camphor.[54] Nicolas Heurteloup in 1794 used musk and cold baths.[55] The standard treatment for tetanus in the Army of the Rhine during 1792–95 was a mixture of two measures of potash in nine to twelve ounces of water and twelve grains of opium during a twenty-four hour period.[56] As palliatives, some of these prescriptions eased the pain of those dying with tetanus, but the nature of the disease remained a mystery.

Fatalities due to gangrene and tetanus were inadvertently encouraged by surgical principles that had been well established prior to 1792. Le Dran's text that recommended quick amputation had been discarded.[57] Bilguer was the most influential opponent of amputation. His monograph, *On the Inutility of the Amputation of Limbs* (1762), had been translated into a number of languages. His principles were championed by the Academy of Surgery, and even Desault favored amputation only as a last resort. Six conditions in which amputation was permissible had been laid down by Bilguer: bad mangling of a limb with death threatening, gangrene, massive contusion and multiple fracture, severe injury to the great arteries, incurable bone decay, and cancer. These rules were based on his compilations of results of peacetime amputations and on the popular "vital forces" theory, which held that a wounded man's reaction to amputation would be critical because of the feeble state of his "vital forces."[58]

Briot thought that these ideas may have been suitable for peacetime surgery but observed that war presented surgeons with entirely different circumstances. They saw limbs partially shot away by artillery, bones splintered by balls, members left hanging by only a few threads of flesh, joints torn and shattered, terrible burns, and massive hemorrhages. A physician had no time to follow rigid procedure when treating ghastly wounds during a retreat or while he was in an exposed position. As Briot said, "The mind did not have time to reason, to calculate probabilities, or to create resources. Experience and coldbloodedness counted for more than talent. Everything had to be done with prompt and decisive action."[59]

Military surgeons were not given the calm and unhurried atmosphere necessary for the task of laboriously picking out bone splinters and bits of clothing from gaping wounds. Locating the open ends of severed arteries and tying them off in the smoke of battle or by flickering candlelight was an enormous problem. There was also the frustration of trying to set and adequately splint a very complicated fracture under battle conditions. Although some wounds did not in themselves dictate amputation, it often had to be done because the patient could not otherwise survive the rigors of transport to the rear.[60]

Nevertheless, Percy's surgical manual, published in 1792, laid down the accepted conservative rules about amputation, and he fought diligently to enforce these rules in his capacity as surgeon-in-chief of the Army of the North and of the Moselle. He complained of having too many "pseudosurgeons who counted their battle actions only by the number of arms and legs they had cut off."[61] Indeed, there were numerous surgeons who fitted the description of the celebrated Lisfranc: "so obsessive a scalpel-wielder that he lamented the passing of the Napoleonic age when the grenadiers had provided him with so many splendid opportunities for amputations."[62]

Conservative practitioners such as Percy, Sabatier, and Lombard favored bone resection, involving the removal of all splinters and foreign particles from a fracture and joining the remaining bone extremities. This was a serious operation that required long treatment and usually resulted in pseudo-arthrosis and functional weakness but it often saved the limb.[63] Bone resections, however, were clinical rarities. The first to excise the head of the humerus and successfully rejoin an arm to the shoulder was Charles White in 1768.[64] The opponents of amputation, with many unprecedented opportunities for experimentation, championed efforts to save limbs by bone resection. Amputation was authorized only if resection failed. As a result, in 1792–93 numerous successful resections were made. Larrey was the first to excise the head of the humerus during the campaign of 1792, although Percy performed the operation successfully many times during the period 1792–95.[65] The first resection of the knee was done by P. F. Moreau (of Bar-sur-Ornans) in 1792, and Percy was credited with helping him.[66] Both Larrey and the Prussian surgeon Goercke resected the elbow joint in 1793. Most surgeons came to prefer resections to amputations in the joint because the tissues at the knee and elbow were not suitable for an adequate flap.[67]

Larrey practiced but did not champion resection. He did his best, in fact, to resist the dogmatic rules on amputation. In this he was bitterly opposed by Percy. Larrey was less concerned with saving limbs than he was with saving men from gangrene and tetanus. He recalled what he had heard surgeons of the War of American Independence say about the advisability of early amputation.[68] He had seen the fatal results of Desault's avoidance of amputation at the time of the Réveillon riots in 1789.[69] In 1792 during the bombardment of Kell, he had seen three volunteers with limbs shattered by exploding shells. They were attended by Simon Boy, who was then a surgeon first class at the Strasbourg hospital. Larrey observed that Boy waited "several days before amputating: not a one [of the wounded men] had the good fortune to recover."[70]

Of the campaigns of 1792 and 1793, Larrey said, "I had carefully observed the phenomena attending gunshot wounds and perceived the advantage of immediate amputation, when the injury required it."[71] At Perpignan, late in 1793, Larrey tried to save two soldiers whose amputations had been delayed seven or eight days, but one died of tetanus and the other of gangrene.[72] Having satisfied himself of the errors of Desault and Percy, Larrey argued for on-the-spot amputation. To him, speed was vital—more vital than technique. Larrey championed his "twenty-four hour" principle, which required the amputation of shattered limbs within that time limit to avoid tetanus and gangrene.[73]

Despite Percy's opposition, Larrey's "twenty-four hour" principle won increasingly widespread acceptance. By 1795, the essentially civilian rules on amputation had been changed by the realities of wartime wounds and of battle surgery. Bone resection was too tedious and difficult for consistent battlefield performance; new guidelines for quick amputation had to be formulated. Five conditions were in effect in 1795 for on-the-spot amputation: (1) shattered bones, (2) limbs partially or completely shot away, (3) much flesh and major arteries missing, even if the bone were sound, (4) muscles, nerves, and small bones too disordered, and (5) when joints were smashed and any hope of movement was gone.[74] There were few major wounds to arms and legs that did not meet at least one of these conditions for quick amputation. Accordingly, Larrey's "twenty-four hour" theory became the rule rather than the exception in French military surgery.[75]

As the rules of amputation were modified to conform to the lessons of wartime, the method of amputation also was adapted from civilian teachings. At first military surgeons observed the old precepts that emphasized technique. Such amputations were slow, done without any anesthesia, and the hot cautery iron was used to seal off severed arteries and veins. The skin flaps were sewn together, the wound covered with ointments, and then bandaged.[76] Leg amputations were often un-satisfactory because the place selected for the incision followed traditional teaching: a point four or five thumb-widths below the knee. This left a conical stump that could be fitted with the commonly used "peg leg." Foot amputation, developed by Chopart, was more satisfactory because his technique left a stump upon which a man could walk; Larrey did this operation frequently.[77] Amputations in the hip joint were rare. This was because there were few occasions for it, not, as Briot said, because French military surgeons "lacked the courage and the coldbloodedness to practice it."[78]

Numerous factors combined to produce the improved amputation technique that military surgeons used in the armies of the First Republic. One was a lack of equipment which forced amputations by pocket knives and ordinary carpenter's saws. Surgeons soon discovered that they secured better drainage and healing when they were without any sutures or needles and were forced simply to hold the flap edges together by a bandage. Another factor was the advent of artificial limbs. In order to adapt the stumps to these new devices, surgeons began making higher incisions when amputating the lower leg. Instead of leaving men with long conical stumps, a cut across the head of the small bone of the leg (the fibula) left a solid, obtuse stump formed by the knee. This new place of amputation resulted in fewer complications and left a far more satisfactory stump.[79]

The amputation techniques employed by Percy, Larrey, and Briot were similar and evidently representative of the procedure most generally used in the armies. Each began with a circular incision through the skin and cellular tissue. Short vertical cuts then enabled an assistant to lift up the skin flaps and turn them back, while the surgeon clipped the membranes that held them to the muscles. Another circular incision cut through the muscles down to the bone and the remaining tissue was split and pulled up so the surgeon could saw through the bone. All veins were then tied off, using threads long enough and lax enough to hold up under the swelling that was to come. The surgeon next trimmed the flesh and skin flaps so that they came back into exact contact. The result was a slightly inverse cone, which needed only a bit of linen to absorb the drainage and an appropriate bandage. Briot preferred to use agglutinative bandages and then to wrap the stump with a large linen bandage.[80]

Larrey's great contribution was his demonstration that two granulating skin surfaces would unite if one was merely laid against the other and the wound was cleaned frequently (today called "union by third intention").[81] He preferred dressing a stump with a soft linen wad, placing two small bandages to form a cross on the end of the stump, and then wrapping the stump with a roller-bandage to keep the flaps together. His technique was especially successful both because of the free drainage allowed by the dressing and because he avoided any salves or ointments which would inhibit drainage. Using only water to wash the wound and changing the bandage from time to time, Larrey revolutionized the treatment of amputees as well as the technique of amputation.[82]

It was a paradox that French surgery and medicine should advance so far during a period when medicines, instruments, supplies, and equipment were so lacking. The exigencies of the early war years forced medical men to improvise, and the emergency conditions of the battlefield permitted experimentation on a scale that was unheard of in peacetime. Many traditional practices and precepts of surgery, often geared to civilian practice, proved to be either erroneous or impossible to follow in wartime. Shortages of equipment and medicines actually promoted advances in wound treatment. Greasy ointments and salves gave way to plain water as the principal treatment for wounds. Larrey originated wound irrigation and popularized the use of moxa. Simple dressings were found to be superior to older, more complicated wrappings. The shortage of supplies and tools made military surgeons masters of the bandage, because it could be substituted for so many peacetime contraptions. The abusive practice of trepanning was discarded, and the treatment of head wounds advanced with its abandonment. The cautery iron fell into disfavor, along with compression, as surgeons learned how to ligate veins and control hemorrhages. In learning how to secure healing by "union of third intention," French military surgeons revolutionized wound treatment.

Experience on the battlefield with a tremendous variety of wounds produced additional advances in military medicine. Wound excision became more selective, shock and stupor in wounded men was better understood, and the old mystery of "wind deaths" was solved. Massive burns received better treatment and beginnings were made in skin grafting and anesthesia. Fewer fatalities occurred when the old temptation to perform battlefield laparotomies was brought under control. Abdominal surgery profited from Sabatier's "playing card technique" in the case of severed intestines, and much abdominal surgery was avoided due to Larrey's teaching of catheterization in cases of bladder injuries. Though gangrene and tetanus were still poorly understood, the conditions that forced surgeons to adopt the principle of immediate amputation led to fewer casualties from these two killers. As amputation was adapted to military requirements, the speed and simpler techniques of the battle surgeons allowed faster and less complicated healing.

Wartime medicine operated under a discipline that forced French physicians and surgeons to abandon many faulty medical practices, damaging operations, and useless medicines. It required them to learn new and better ways of healing and learn them quickly. In civilian life, such progress would have been quite impossible in so short a time. The war that began in 1792 helped to trigger a profound medical revolution. Its battlefields became medical schools because formal medicine and surgical training no longer existed in France. Of course, the battlefield had always been a training ground for French military surgeons, but few had ever seen anything like the bloody engagements fought by mass armies at Fleurus, Jemappes, Hondeschoot, and Wattignies. Numberless cadavers were at hand for autopsy and dissection, and the national emergency required of surgeons quick improvisation and audacity in trying to care for the casualties of battle. The lessons learned by surgeons during 1792, 1793, and 1794 produced significant modifications in French medicine when the National Convention finally revived formal medical education in 1795.

NOTES

1. Briot, *Chirurgie militaire*, p.181.
2. Quoted in Laignel-Lavastine, *Histoire générale* 3: 10.
3. Delorme, *War Surgery*, pp.21, 113.
4. Briot, *Chirurgie militaire*, p.41.
5. Ganges, *Représentants du peuple* 1: 401.
6. Briot, *Chirurgie militaire*, p.381.
7. Briot dossier, carton BII 204, Val-de-Grâce.
8. Acq. fran. III, 21a, pp.27–30, Archives nationales.
9. Conseil de Santé documents, carton 11, Arch. hist. Service de Santé.
10. Briot, *Chirurgie militaire*, p.99; Laurent, *Percy*, pp.298, 301.
11. Briot dossier, carton BII 204, Val-de-Grâce.
12. Ibid.; Briot, *Chirurgie militaire*, pp.91–92.
13. Briot dossier, carton BII 204, Val-de-Grâce.
14. Ibid.
15. Lorentz dossier, carton 209/1, ibid.; Percy dossier, carton 211 bis, ibid.; Conseil de Santé documents, carton 12, Arch. hist. Service de Santé.

16. Conseil de Santé documents, carton 12, Arch. hist. Service de Santé.

17. Applied to the skin and ignited, the moxa served to produce a scab or acted as a counter-irritant (Japanese: *moe kusa*, burning herbs). See Jones, Hoerr and Osol, *Blakiston's New Gould Medical Dictionary*, p.642.

18. Larrey, *Surgical Essays*, pp.24—27. Percy liked to use a moxa made from the common sunflower. When ignited, it smelled something like coffee. See *Dict. encyclopédique sci. méd.*, 4th ser., 12: 591.

19. Larrey, *Recueil des mémoires*, pp.4—13; *Dictionnaire de médecine* 20: 296—99.

20. The moxa was introduced into the Far East and Europe from ancient Egypt. Jones, Hoerr and Osol, *Blakiston's Medical Dictionary*, p.642.

21. Percy dossier, carton 211 bis, Val-de-Graĉe.

22. Conseil de Santé documents, carton 11, Arch. hist. Service de Santé.

23. Briot, *Chirurgie militaire*, p.385.

24. Briot dossier, carton BII 204, Val-de-Grâce; Garrison, *Notes*, p.152. The adhesive bandage could be applied dry or treated with some medicinal or antiseptic and then plastered on the patient.

25. Briot, *Chirurgie militaire*, pp.17—18, 380.

26. "La découverte de l'anesthésie chirurgicale pour la reduction des luxations par des rebouteurs au XVIIIe siècle," *Archives provinciales de chirurgie* 20: 611.

27. Ibid.; Guillaume, *Convention* 3: 229.

28. Thorwald, *Century of the Surgeon*, p.9.

29. Conseil de Santé documents, carton 11, Arch. hist. Service de Santé; Laurent, *Percy*, pp.6—7; *Dict. encyclopedique sci. méd.*, 2d ser., 1: 123; 21: 647.

30. Boy dossier, carton 204 B/1, Val-de-Grâce.

31. Briot dossier, carton BII 204, ibid.

32. Acq. fran. III, 21a, pp.27—30, Archives nationales.

33. Larrey, *Memoirs* 1: 44—45. Larrey taught the use of ointment of styrax once suppuration began and nitrate of silver when granulations rose above the lips of the wound. He rejected Hippocrates's insistence upon a low diet for burn victims and gave them conventional meals.

34. Pelletan dossier, carton 212, Val-de-Grâce.

35. Briot, *Chirurgie militaire*, pp.29—30.

36. Briot dossier, carton BII 204, Val-de-Grâce; Desault dossier, carton 206, ibid.; Lombard dossier, carton 209/1, ibid.

37. Larrey, *Memoirs* 1: 31.

38. Briot, *Chirurgie militaire*, p.124.

39. Ibid., p.125.

40. Petit, *Treatise on Diseases of the Bones*, pp.4ff.

41. Briot dossier, carton BII 204, Val-de-Grâce.

42. Conseil de Santé documents, carton 12, Arch. hist. Service de Santé.

43. P. Bonnette, "Rapport médicale sur la blessure du générale Marceau," *Chron. méd.* 17: 79.

44. Briot, *Chirurgie militaire*, p.132.

45. Laparotomy: major surgery in the abdominal cavity involving an incision through the peritoneum.

46. Conseil de Santé documents, carton 12, Arch. hist. Service de Santé.

47. Sabatier dossier, carton 213, Val-de-Grâce.

48. Briot, *Chirurgie militaire*, p.45.

49. Conseil de Santé documents, carton 11, Arch. hist. Service de Santé.

50. Briot, *Chirurgie militaire*, pp.243, 265.

51. Ibid., pp. 242, 247–48, 255.

52. Percy dossier, carton 211 bis, Val-de-Grâce.

53. Jean Jacques Canin (1769–1836), Canin dossier, carton 205, ibid.; Claude Barthélemy Jean Leclerc (1762–1808), Leclerc dossier, carton 209/1, ibid.; Briot, *Chirurgie militaire*, pp.241-48.

54. Lombard dossier, carton 209/1, Val-de-Grâce; Lorentz dossier, carton 209/1, ibid.

55. Acq. fran. III, 21a, pp.27–30, Archives nationales.

56. Briot dossier, carton BII 204, Val-de-Grâce.

57. Henri François Le Dran, *Traité ou reflexions tirées de la pratique sur les playes d'armes à feu* (Paris, 1737).

58. Briot, *Chirurgie militaire*, p.76; Garrison, *Notes*, p.153.

59. Briot, *Chirurgie militaire*, p.203.

60. Conseil de Santé documents, carton 11, Arch. hist. Service de Santé.

61. Percy, *Manuel du chirurgien d'armée* (Paris, 1792); Laurent, *Percy*, pp.252–54.

62. Thorwald, *Century of the Surgeon*, p.7.

63. Lombard dossier, carton 209/1, Val-de-Grâce; Percy dossier, carton 211 bis, ibid.; Sabatier dossier, carton 213, ibid.

64. Garrison, *Notes*, p.153. The head of the humerus (upper arm bone) joins the arm to the shoulder at the joint.

65. Larrey, *Memoirs* 1: 34.

66. Laignel-Lavastine, *Histoire générale* 3: 98.

67. Garrison, *Notes* p.153.

68. Da Costa, "Larrey," *Johns Hopkins Hosp. Bull.* 17: 207.

69. Larrey, *Memoirs* 1: 18–19.

70. Larrey, *Relation historique*, p.339.

71. Larrey, *Memoirs* 1: 31.

72. Larrey, *Relation historique*, p.339. His brother, François, was a surgeon first-class at Perpignan's Hospital Brutus. Ibid., p.389.

73. Larrey, *Memoirs* 1: 31; Laignel-Lavastine, *Histoire générale* 3: 8−9.

74. Briot, *Chirurgie militaire*, p.191.

75. Larrey, *Memoirs* 1: 31; Laignel-Lavastine, *Histoire générale* 3: 8. Recognizing that, with no anesthesia, an amputation ought not last over four minutes, Larrey regularly cut off legs in less than a minute. By 1808, he could amputate an arm in seventeen seconds.

76. Da Costa, "Larrey," *Johns Hopkins Hosp. Bull.* 17: 207.

77. Larrey, *Memoirs* 1: 34.

78. Briot, *Chirurgie militaire*, p.182.

79. Ibid., p. 184; Bottet, "Le passé," *Cauducée 5: 153.*

80. Descriptions of individual amputation techniques may be found in Larrey, *Relation historique*, pp.373−76; Briot, *Chirurgie militaire*, pp.204−5; and Laurent, *Percy*, pp.262−65.

81. Da Coste, "Larrey," *Johns Hopkins Hosp. Bull.* 17: 207, 213.

82. Ibid.

Chapter Eight

HOSPITALS AND THE NEW MEDICINE

The mass casualties suffered by the armies necessitated a search for more facilities in which to house and care for them. The National Convention began moving many old veterans out of the Invalides in Paris during January of 1793 and authorized the reception of wounded soldiers. The old monastery of Val-de-Grâce on the Rue St. Jacques was studied by Coste and Bayen, then reopened and prepared as a military hospital. By July 31, it began operating under a War Ministry decree. With a capacity of 1,000 to 1,200 patients, Val-de-Grâce was originally intended to relieve overcrowding at the Gros-Caillou and to serve the sick men of the Paris garrison. However, the flow of sick and wounded from the battlefronts immediately doubled, and soon tripled, the number of patients the Val-de-Grâce had to serve. To relieve some of the strain, medical authorities undertook the segregation of men according to their ailments; those with the itch and venereal disease were sent to the Saint-Denis or to the Hôpital du Midi, which specialized in the treatment of venerals. The Midi, the Hôtel-Dieu, and the Charité were expanded, and studies were undertaken in late 1793 that were to convert the St. Louis into a hospital for skin diseases and two other old monasteries, the St. Antoine and Port Royal (the Maternité), into hospitals by 1795.[1]

Throughout France, this process of conversion and expansion of hospital facilities characterized the year 1793. Urgent wartime demands, especially the shortage of medical men and the huge numbers of sick and wounded, sharply reversed the prerevolutionary trend away from hospitals. Now the hospitals were proving to be the only efficient way to try to cope with the military casualties of 1792—93 and attempt to satisfy the demands of the Revolution for improved public health care. Now that medical teaching in the universities and the military ampitheatres had been abolished, hospitals became the only logical place for instruction in medicine, surgery, and pharmacy. Here, too, the new emphasis upon observation, examination, diagnosis, statistics, and autopsy could be implemented most effectively. Consequently, the hospital reform movement of the 1780s had regained much of its momentum by 1793. The Revolution's goal had changed from earlier cries for the abolition of hospitals. The emerging concept was that of strengthened and improved hospitals to serve as the core of medicine, not only for diagnosis and treatment of the sick and disabled but also for medical instruction and research.

The critical problem of epidemic diseases in the armies of the French Republic is illustrated by the fact that "fevers" was a standard category that led all other classifications of disability, even running ahead of "wounds" by ratios of two-to-one and three-to-one. From original reports filed with the Council of Health during the winter of 1792—93 by selected representative military hospitals,[2] the pattern of disabilities was evident.

Date	Hospital	Fevers	Wounded	Itch	Venereal	Totals
26 Nov. '92	Dunkerque	99	67	20	81	303*
28 Nov. '92	Berguere	57	31	26	11	139**
10 Dec. '92	Tournai	91	36	9	9	145
6 Jan. '93	Maubeuge	258	100	17	14	389
6 Jan. '93	Mons	63	35	12	7	117
17 Jan. '93	Brussels	553	156	304	163	1116
7 Feb. '93	Aix-la-Chapelle	309	62			371
7 Feb. '93	Namur	130	40			170
3 Mar. '93	Thionville	192	57			249

(* includes 36 undiagnosed; ** includes 14 undiagnosed)

In all of these hospitals, troops with wounds constituted, on the average, about 22 percent of the patients. On the other hand, as winter came on the incidence of fever soared. Expressed in terms of percentages, fever cases in these hospitals rose from 23 percent in November to nearly 80 percent in February and March, 1793.

Of course, "fevers" was an extremely elastic term, covering meningitis, malaria, typhus, typhoid fever, pneumonia, scurvy, late stages of dysentery and tetanus, advanced cases of hospital gangrene, and various intermittent, low-grade fevers. The swelling load of fever cases coincided with the cold, wet weather of December, January, and February. Also noticeable was the enormous upsurge of itch and venereal disease as French soldiers moved into Belgium. After January, 1793, the fever epidemics left few places in the hospitals for troops with less serious ailments, and undiagnosed cases tended to go unreported, being lumped with "fevers" in later reports. The frustration and desperation of physicians trying to cope with the flood of fever victims was summarized in a report dated May 15 from Nancy: "The weather is cold and humid. There is not much improvement in those with fever and we have tried everything." The response of the Council of Health was reassuring: "The winds will soon shift to south and southeast—then you will see improvement."[3]

Soaring mortality rates starkly revealed the helplessness of physicians in dealing with epidemic fevers. Traditionally, they fought them with emetics, laxatives, and bleedings. Although the following figures are from reports of different hospitals over a four-month period, the mortality rates for fever patients are significant.[4] They show consistently high death rates from "fevers" and help explain the frantic concern of physicians, generals, and politicians.

Date	Hospital	Fever Patients	Died	Mortality Rate
26 Nov. '92	Dunkerque	99	26	1 out of 4
28 Nov. '92	Berguere	57	14	1 out of 4
10 Dec. '92	Tournai	91	18	1 out of 5
6 Jan. '93	Maubeuge	258	78	1 out of 4
6 Jan. '93	Mons	63	19	1 out of 3
17 Jan. '93	Brussels	553	138	1 out of 4
7 Feb. '93	Aix-la-Chapelle	309	44	1 out of 7
7 Feb. '93	Naumur	130	19	1 out of 7
3 Mar. '93	Thionville	192	19	1 out of 10

There were no "typical" approaches to or treatments of "fevers" because physicians disagreed on both cause and diagnosis. However, a report by the physician Jean Jomard from Mayence early in 1793 is illustrative of one viewpoint: Jomard attributed the fever epidemic in the Army of the Rhine to housing soldiers in humid barracks during the winter, "with little ventilation, the stale air prompts a putrid miasma and, when you add to that the bad quality of the majority of soldiers, you find the cause soon enough." After detailing the symptoms of typhoid fever, Jomard described his treatment: "Although bleeding seems to help the inflammation temporarily by improving circulation, if the fever persists give a second bleeding, less than the first; I have rarely seen the need of a third. If the putrid fever resists prescribed treatments after 8–10 days, we purge the patients and give them sweetened barley water mixed with reddened alcohol, bathe the legs and abdomen with alcohol solutions— such are the means that I have used with the best success."[5]

Despite the best efforts of some truly able practitioners, the prestige of the average military physician continued to be eroded during 1793. Complaints of ignorance leveled against them by surgeons, especially the outspoken Percy, and charges of laxity, incompetence, and treason brought by representatives on mission were increasingly heard. Another factor contributing to this process was the crucial shortage of medicinals. During the early months of 1793, the Council of Health was overwhelmed by hundreds of urgent requisitions and pleas for medicines and supplies for the hospitals.[6] Exotic prescription ingredients which characterized the secret remedies of physicians were no longer readily available, and military physicians were forced to simpler treatments devised from what was on hand. Required to work with only a few basic medicinals, physicians could offer a patient no better prescription than could surgeons and pharmacists. With respect to surgeons, the physicians also found themselves less useful both in the hospitals and on the battlefield, because the surgeons had an indispensable skill.

Still another aspect of the growing general disenchantment with military physicians was their obvious inability to understand and to cope with epidemic diseases. Battlefield medicine was more often than not the true province of the surgeon, who was not generally held responsible for epidemics. Yet their simpler procedures and prescriptions for diseases during this period had produced results that impressed pragmatic political and military authorities. Consequently, despite the favored status of physicians and their traditional attitudes of superiority, wartime epidemics overwhelmed them, and the gap between physicians and surgeons closed and disappeared in the military service. This is the real significance of the circular letter from Gautier, Assistant War Minister, dated February 11, 1793, and addressed to all hospital personnel: "The replacement of physicians which hospitals and the armies have lost, whether by illness, death or other reason, cannot take place promptly due to the emergency. So the Minister has decided that in these cases the duties of physicians will be temporarily taken over by the surgeons-in-chief."[7]

More and more during 1793 surgeons took over fever cases, and the contrast in treatments by physicians and surgeons became sharper. Percy attributed the high death rate from typhus to the medicines administered by the physicians. While the military doctors were still trying to prescribe their individual secret remedies, surgeons who scorned exotic medicinals were securing good survival rates through simple isolation, good food, and rest.[8] Percy was no unbiased reporter, being contemptuous of physicians, but many surgeons were reporting similar results. Lafont-Gouzi recalled that one soldier came to him in the eighth day of such a fever, "after having been bled, and several times evacuated both high and low" by physicians. Prescribing a little laudanum, milk, and rest, Lafont-Gouzi declared that he effected a cure.[9]

The dysentery that commonly afflicted the armies was scarcely less destructive than the typhus. While the army veterinarians under Lafosse were saving horses affected by it, Percy charged that "military physicians were still killing people with their 'incendiary' prescriptions."[10] Percy regarded dysentery as an internal inflammation, and though the common practice was to treat it with stimulants, he taught the use of small doses of ipecacuanha.[11] Coste was a far more accomplished epidemologist than Percy. Struggling against centuries of medical tradition, he tried to teach, persuade, or coerce his army physicians to adopt simpler and better ways. He knew that scurvy came from a lack of fruits and vegetables, and for measles and smallpox he urged vaccination. For dealing with fevers, he put great stock in simple quinine and sought to prevent dysentery by watching the food people ate and the water they drank. He agreed with Percy that small doses of powdered ipecacuanha was the best prescription for dysentery.[12]

The frustration of Coste and Percy's anger was understandable when the Metz physician Michael Tennetar rushed into print with his booklet on the treatment of dysentery. Tennetar listed seventeen different remedies one could try. Powdered ipecacuanha, Arabian gum, rhubarb, terebinthe, calomel, and quinquina are all key items in these prescriptions, but their pattern was that of the traditional emetics, laxatives, and bleedings. "And here is another purgative which has been widely used in these circumstances," Tennetar wrote, urging a calomel-based laxative for the treatment of dysentery.[13]

Hospital gangrene was endemic in all hospital facilities, and few wounded men escaped its ravages. Among the health officers there was no agreement as to the nature of this disease, and the methods of dealing with it varied widely. Lafont-Gouzi recognized hospital gangrene as the major cause of relapses in patients and thought it spread through the use of the common drinking cup in hospitals, though he attributed its source to bad food.[14] P. F. Moreau viewed it as a contagious disease that attacked the nerves, while Briot rejected contagion and classified it with dysentery and scurvy. Percy did not think it was contagious and believed it to result from sharp fluctuations in temperature.[15]

The common wartime remedies attempted for gangrene were lemon juice, vinegar, spirits of camphor, and charcoal. On bad infections, caustics such as nitrate of silver, nitrate of mercury, and muriate of antimony, were used. Percy bathed all wounds with lemon juice or vinegar when changing the dressings, hoping to control hospital gangrene in this way.[16] Because most medical men were only treating the symptoms of this highly contagious disease and were ignoring the very elementary sanitary precautions, hospital gangrene continued to ravage the wounded. It sapped the strength of the armies by turning slight wounds into open, festering areas that condemned the wounded to long, slow periods of recuperation.

As the medical situation worsened in the summer and fall of 1793, figures from reports covering the period from June to November, 1793, at two big military hospitals, Landau and Metz,[17] illustrate the magnitude of the crisis.

	Landau					Metz				
	On Hand	In	Out	Dead	Carry Over	On Hand	In	Out	Dead	Carry Over
June 1793										
Fevers	339	894	801	64	368	626	863	780	81	628
Wounded	70	32	34	4	64	213	414	332	12	283
Venereals	12	24	18		18	91	89	135		45
Itch	7	11	9		9	82	130	166		46
				68					93	
July 1793										
Fevers	368	903	965	97	209	628	1668	1504	61	731
Wounded	64	104	32	15	121	283	436	500	10	209
Venereals	18	31	12		12	46	42	26		62
Itch	9	15	12		12	46	42	26		62
				112					71	
August 1793										
Fevers	209	1326	790	88	693	731	1726	1595	71	791
Wounded	121	119	102	18	120	209	937	919	11	216
Venereals	20	33	27	1	25	42	36	31		47
Itch	12	18	13		17	62	56	62		56
				107					82	
September 1793										
Fevers	693	811	770	191	583	791	730	850	107	564
Wounded	120	128	193	6	89	216	232	299	6	143
Venereals	25	36	29	1	31	47	98	46	1	98
Itch	17	4	18		3	56	230	166		120
				198					114	
October 1793										
Fevers	583	617	705	142	353	564	831	720	92	583
Wounded	89	111	136	8	56	143	319	195	5	262
Venereals	31	6	27		10	98	118	99	1	116
Itch	3		3			120	141	139		122
				150					98	

The comparatively low mortality rate of those patients with wounds illustrates the advantage that surgeons were gaining over physicians. Fever victims were dying at very high rates and in great numbers compared to the toll taken by wounds.

	Landau			Metz		
	Number	*Deaths*	*Rate*	*Number*	*Deaths*	*Rate*
Fever Cases						
June, 1793	1,233	64	1/20	1,489	81	1/18
July	1,271	97	1/13	2,296	61	1/38
August	1,535	88	1/18	1,457	71	1/34
September	1,504	142	1/8	1,521	107	1/15
October	1,200	142	1/8	1,395	92	1/15
Wounded						
June, 1793	102	4	1/25	627	12	1/52
July	168	15	1/11	719	10	1/72
August	240	18	1/13	1,146	11	1/104
September	248	6	1/41	448	6	1/75
October	200	8	1/25	462	5	1/92

The climax of the summer fever epidemics appeared in the actual fatalities and in the high ratio of deaths in September and October. The lower death rates at Metz resulted from at least two factors: The Metz hospital was still one of the best military medical facilities in France, and Metz could assign hopeless fever patients to satellite facilities and concentrate upon saving those remaining. This was evident in the September report from Metz: "Our critical periods have been frequent. We cannot give an exact accounting because we have sent many of those with fevers and gangrene to the ambulances."[18] Landau, on the other hand, was a makeshift forward hospital which suffered more critical shortages of medicines and medical men, and tended to keep fever and wound victims while assigning those with the itch and venereal disease to facilities in the rear. This policy resulted in forward facilities like Landau showing almost none of these cases by the end of October and others like Metz filling more and more places with venereals and troops with the itch. Specifically, from a peak of 61 venereals in September, Landau admitted only 6 in October and only 10 remained in the hospital by the end of the month. The last three itch patients were discharged during October. Metz, meanwhile, achieved October peaks in both categories: 216 venereals and 261 with the itch.[19]

The main problem with these cases did not lie in confusion and disagreement over diagnosis or treatment. Mercury pills for venereals were standard (guaicum when the mercury ran out) and iron or zinc sulfide were generally prescribed for the itch. However, venereals were lost to action for at least 40 days and those with the itch for a minimum of three weeks. The critical shortages of medicinals posed the principal obstacle to returning men to duty even after these periods. In the fall of 1793, they could not be treated properly and, if permitted, remained in the hospitals and clogged these facilities along with fever patients and the wounded.

As the idea of hospital medicine developed out of revolutionary thought and wartime necessity, the Convention moved steadily to increase subsidies to hospitals, to standardize and centralize their operations, and to try to improve the quality of health care. In the fall of 1793, the Committee of Public Safety distributed to all health officers an *Instruction on the Means of Preserving Sanitation and Purifying the Air in Rooms in the Military Hospitals of the Republic*. This brochure reflected, to some extent, the Committee's awareness of the need to inform the ill-trained medical men who were being drafted. It also revealed what was considered to be up-to-date methods, even though the instructions given showed little recognition of the desperate situations encountered by medical men in the field hospitals.[20]

The new rules specified that patients entering hospitals were to have their hands and feet washed in sterile water, and their cloaks and clothes were to be beaten and given a sulphur fumigation. Beds were to be located away from the walls, with two to three feet between them, and mattress straw was to be changed, beaten, and restuffed every six months. There were to be sufficient toilets (*chaises percées*) for all patients, and they were to be kept near the men needing them most. Water was to be kept in these toilets, and they were to be washed after each use and smeared with a strong desiccative oil. All urinals were to be emptied as soon as possible. Wooden beds were to be painted or varnished, the floors and walls whitewashed, and all tables and chairs washed daily with a strong alkaline solution. Fans were prescribed for moving the air around and, when the heat was the worst, physicians were required to place tree branches and potted plants around to refresh the air. Daily fumigations were specified, using hydrochloric, muriatic, or sulphuric acids, and strong disinfectants were recommended. Curiously, nothing was said about changing the bed linens or an occasional fumigation of blankets. However, some recognition of the shortage of medical equipment was evident in the Convention's subsequent warning to military surgeons not to leave their instruments in a room where any muriatic acid vapors were, because the reaction would rust them instantly.[21] Alarmed by the spreading epidemic illnesses, the Committee of Public Safety issued subsequent hospital regulations, such as its idealistic decree of November 15, 1793, requiring that every hospital patient be given a private bed and that all beds be separated from each other by a distance of three feet.[22]

Just as the exigencies of 1793 had tended to equalize physicians, surgeons, and pharmacists into "health officers," also in process was the reunion of medicine and surgery after centuries of separation. A number of prerevolutionary developments had pointed in this direction, including the growing rejection of philosophical "systems" and the beginning of clinical medicine. The emergence of the hospital as a medical center, the search for the cause of epidemic diseases in the war years from 1792 to 1796, and the ideology of the Revolution itself—each in its own way was a powerful stimulant to the development of a new medicine.

The old Hippocratic notion of the climatic causes of disease lingered in the beliefs of some physicians that the first frost produced conjunctivitis or that the change of seasons somehow affected epidemic fevers. Others, including Hallé and Tourtelle, shared Rousseau's opinion that it was civilization that undermined human health and increased the incidence of disease.[23] Reinforced by a literary legacy that extolled the "noble savage" unspoiled by civilization, this naive view imagined native settings where disease was unknown. In both of these approaches to epidemology, there was a core of fatalism; because no one could control the climate and few Frenchmen were inclined to give up their civilized society, disease was inevitable.

The Revolution could not accept these approaches, especially in a time of crisis and of vast epidemic illnesses. Two other theories of mass disease could be considered: contagionism and social causation. The somewhat vague notions of Fourcroy, Alibert, and Moreau of a contagious "virus" were never well developed. Provincial physicians who advanced the idea of contagion, such as Pierre Bretonneau, were of no influence in Paris, and anyone who spoke energetically of the idea of microscopic living parasites risked being labeled "absurd" or "medieval" in his thinking.[24] It was just too difficult, before pathogenic microorganisms and their carriers (like Typhoid Mary or mosquitoes) were known, to prove contagion. Besides, the idea of contagion was associated with the vested interests that feudal bureaucrats had had in quarantines. A theory of medicine thus tainted with memories of the Old Regime bore too great a handicap.

On the other hand, a "social thoery of disease" harmonized more neatly with revolutionary ideology and its goals. The miserable economic and social conditions of the people could account for epidemic diseases.

Influential ideologues, such as the liberal physicians Cabanis and Guillotin, had expounded this thesis, and similar opinions were voiced by laymen as well as the Jacobin doctors in the national assemblies. Proper social reforms could control disease and, after all, social reform was at the center of the Revolution. There was even a corollary to this social causation theory, vigorously advanced by some, including Chaussier: "If disease had social causes, if the state of freedom is the best social state, health should also be best under freedom."[25] This idea meshed with the hopes and expectations of the French people, as expressed in the *cahiers* and in subsequent demands for the amelioration of the condition of the poor and for better public health care. So, the physicians of the Revolution increasingly tended to embrace a "filth-miasma" approach to disease. If the root cause of epidemic illnesses lay in squalor and foul living and working conditions, both contagionists and social causationists could still press for better conditions. This approach to medicine was readily linked with the will to reform and a basic belief in progress.

The reforming energy of the filth-miasma concept was augmented by the work of many medical men, most of whom were catapulted into places of prominence and influence by the Revolution and its wars. As civilian clinicians or as military health officers, they were hospital-oriented and believed in the value of experience and observation. Autopsies, statistics, and case histories were the raw materials out of which they sought to construct a new and superior understanding of the cause and cure of disease.

One of the valuable contributions to a new medicine was the massive flow of hospital reports to the various authorities in Paris during the war years. Whether submitted by medical officers to the War Ministry or to the Council of Health or by political agents to the Committee of Public Safety, these documents provided statistical information and detailed descriptions of health conditions on a scale hitherto unimagined. Information on types of wounds and how they were inflicted, on types of diseases, disability periods, mortality and survival rates, medicinals requested (as well as those gradually being discarded), supplies and equipment needed, inventories of all hospital furnishings, and medical personnel records were significant items all available for study and analysis by medical men at various levels of authority. Wartime necessity and centralized power in Paris during the Terror and afterwards made it possible to attempt the standardization of medicine and surgery, requiring the application of what was thought to be the best approaches, procedures, equipment, and medicinals.

Of even greater value was the variety of memoranda, special studies, and autopsy reports written during the war years by military physicians and surgeons. Most were handwritten and submitted to the Council of Health, although some were actually published. The quality of these reports was very uneven, but the great quantity of them suggests three important developments. First, epidemic illnesses were of such staggering proportions that the resignation of the past had to be discarded in favor of a vigorous search for new theories, more accurate disease classifications, better treatments, and even ideas of prevention. Second, a changing approach to medicine based upon observation and experience was gradually spreading among French medical men as increasingly they utilized statistics, compiled thousands of case studies, and painstakingly prepared autopsy reports. Third, there was a growing tendency for an individual physician or surgeon, recognizing the magnitude and the variety of illnesses, to concentrate his interest upon one category of disability.

A great many civilian clinicians, in Paris and elsewhere, should be mentioned because of their active role in influencing medical change during this period. However, specific reference to three of the most famous will suffice to show important new attitudes and values: P. J. Desault, Philippe Pinel, and J. M. Corvisart. Desault has appropriately been labeled "the last great surgeon of the old school and the first great surgeon of the new."[26] His introduction of clinical teaching at the Hôtel-Dieu was innovative, and his influence extended to Pinel and Corvisart, to his students—Boyer, Larrey, and Bichat, and to others too numerous to mention here. As Owsei Temkin has observed, "Through his pupils and through the example of his clinical teaching, Desault emerges as the man from whom the Paris school derived more inspiration than anyone else."[27] Desault had no peer as an example of the value of exact observation and as an advocate of the relation of surgery to its anatomical basis, and the new medicine of the 1790s owed much to his genius.

Philippe Pinel is remembered primarily for his psychiatric work, but his contemporaries knew him as a great teacher and systematizer in the field of internal medicine. A moderate revolutionary, he was appointed as a physician at the Bicêtre in August, 1793, where his intelligent treatment of the insane attracted wide attention. A friend of Condorcet, Cabanis, and Franklin, Pinel was a genuine *philosophe* of the eighteenth century, so much so that his most famous medical works were entitled *Nosographie philosophique* (1798) and *Medicophilosophical Treatise on Mental Illness* (1801). Representing over a decade of labor, these books show Pinel's desertion of Hippocrates, his five new disease classifications, and hundreds of documented case histories. Pinel opposed bleeding and purging and favored innoculation and vaccination. He believed in the value of observation and insisted that medical studies should be started in a hospital. One of the originators of clinical instruction, Pinel was a firm advocate of the value of statistics and felt that autopsies and autopsy records were essential parts of medical practice. The influence of his ideas was felt by those who worked with him during his years at the Bicêtre (1793), at the new Ecole de Santé (1794), and at the Charité (1795).[28]

There was another important clinician at the Charité, the great diagnostician and heart specialist, J. N. Corvisart. Strongly opposed to philosophical theories of medicine, he pioneered pathological anatomy, and his *Diseases of the Heart* (1806) was packed with case histories gathered over many years. Every patient he lost was autopsied. Corvisart popularized and excelled in the use of percussion, the palpation technique that opened the door for better diagnosis in chest diseases. Like Pinel and Desault, he practiced "expectant" medicine, rejecting the massive use of medicinals in favor of a confidence in the healing capacity of the human body when an ailment was properly diagnosed and specifically treated. Corvisart made the Charité a center of clinical teaching and furthered the concept of the hospital as the proper setting in which medical teaching and health care should be conducted.[29]

While the Paris clinicians were important contributors, the new medicine owed as much to a host of military medical men during this period. Coste, Percy, Desgenettes, Larrey, Lombard, Boy, and Briot are well known, but there were other equally representative figures in the area of military medicine. Pierre Coze, with the Army of the Rhine, in 1792 published a *Mémoire sur la fièvre pretechicale nerveuse qui a régne en Alsace pendant l'hiver de 1791* (a type of typhus or perhaps meningitis). In 1793, he produced a study of scurvy. Both of these works were filled with detailed descriptions of symptoms, the progress of the diseases, and the results of the autopsies and chemical analyses upon which Coze always insisted.[30] Similar epidemological studies were done by L. Boudenot on diarrhea (1794) and on low-grade fevers (1794),[31] and by Jean Jomard on typhoid fever (1793) and on intermittent fevers (1794).[32] Both Demours and Guérin produced detailed works on epidemic ophthalmia in 1793, suggesting filth as its cause (rather than climate!) and contact as its mode of transmission.[33]

One of the most complete and patiently detailed studies was Louis Philippe Dupont's massive report on the hospitals around Mayence during the siege of 1793. The results of forced improvisations in medicine and surgery, full statistical data, complete autopsy reports, and Dupont's own insights based upon his experience and observation made his work a model for others.[34] Tempiez, physician-in-chief at Colmar, prepared a thorough study of pulmonary diseases based upon his observations during the winters of 1793 and 1794.[35] Briot, who became a believer in "expectant" medicine, won recognition for his work on abdominal wounds.[36] Larrey wrote brilliantly and persuasively on tetanus and gangrene, supporting his conclusions with overwhelming statistics and autopsy reports.[37] Along with Larrey, Charles Louis Dumas and Claude Leclerc were military anatomical-pathologists who furnished Paris with a steady stream of autopsy reports on virtually every conceivable type of mortality.[38]

Although these men tended to specialize in their areas of knowledge, 'the development of true medical specialties is not involved here. As George Rosen has already indicated, "The development of medical specialization derives not so much from an extensive accumulation of specialized factual knowledge, but rather from a conception of disease which permits an intensive application to certain circumscribed problem areas."[39]

What is of paramount importance is the evidence in all of these wartime studies that a new concept of disease was indeed evolving and that it reflected the consequence of close cooperation between military physicians and surgeons. For a long time, surgeons had had to rely upon physical signs in their diagnoses. Tumors, abscesses, ulcers, wounds, broken bones, or gangrene could be seen or felt. In cases of aneurysm, hernia, or cataract, a localized structural change had first to be visualized before operating. So the surgeons studied anatomy because they had to know both normal and abnormal human structure. Physicians, on the other hand, traditionally scorned anatomy and remained much too ignorant of it. There were symptoms to be explained but this could be done by a speculative pathology which referred to humors, vital juices, acrimonies, or irritability increases. When the Revolution tended to equalize and unite physicians and surgeons as "health officers" and they found themselves involved together in caring for fevers, wounds, skin diseases, scurvy, and the removal of foreign objects, the physicians began to drop their speculative theories and adopt the surgico-anatomical point of view. The causes of illness, as autopsies came to be routine, could be seen as tumors, abscesses, ulcers, hemorrhages and inflammations inside the body.[40]

While it is true that a number of the great clinicians of the prerevolutionary period were pathological anatomists and through them medicine and surgery were slowly being reunited, the war years of 1792–95 vastly accelerated this process. With great numbers of average medical practitioners pressed into military service, there was an unparalleled opportunity and, indeed, necessity for them to become anatomists. The physician, in fact, found himself increasingly at a disadvantage after 1792 unless he changed his concepts; he did not possess the surgeon's special skill, and he found the surgeon more than willing to prescribe for and care for his patients. Losing prestige, forced to rely upon simple medicinals, overwhelmed by epidemic illnesses, and spurred by both political representatives and aggressive and inventive surgeons, the physician had every incentive to adopt the surgeon's view and embrace a localized pathology. This is a key development in French medicine that has been outlined by Owsei Temkin in his brilliant study of the role of surgery in the rise of modern medical thought: "It is hardly possible to claim that the medical reform came first, the stimulus to surgery afterwards . . . . Surgery, for many centuries, had relied upon an objective anatomical diagnosis. In turning to a localized pathology, medicine adopted a point of view prevalent among surgeons . . . . Because the reorientation of medicine took place within a relatively short period and led to dramatic results in diagnosis and nosology, it has impressed us more than the steady advance of surgery."[41]

While the influence of the clinical teaching of Desault, Pinel, and Corvisart upon their friends and students was strong and pervasive, the work of many other clinicians was important in the change. Even the accumulated influence of many clinicians could not provide the set of conditions that the Revolution and the war furnished for the rapid and widespread development of a more modern medicine. Revolutionary ideology demanded medical reform and the equality of physicians and surgeons, and it pushed hard for a concept of medicine that aimed at eliminating disease through the improvement of filthy conditions. In seeking improved public health care and better means of treating a staggering number of wartime wounds and epidemic diseases, the Revolution seized upon the hospital as the key medical institution for both healing and teaching. The war's mass casualties and mounting epidemics actually gave the surgeon a temporary ascendancy over the physician. In the course of the period from 1792 to 1795, the case studies, statistics, and plentiful cadavers made anatomists of hundreds of average physicians through the autopsies that surgeons demanded and performed. Only in a period of crisis and war could the conditions have been produced for a new medicine accepted, voluntarily or under duress, by such great numbers of medical men. This is why the reorientation of French medicine came so swiftly and so thoroughly after the reestablishment of formal medical training and the end of the war in 1795.

NOTES

1. Laws and Decrees, carton 1, Arch. hist. Service de Santé; Rieux and Hassenforder, *Histoire*, p.23.

2. Army hospitals, cartons 25, 28, 29, 30, Arch. hist. Service de Santé. Scores of similar reports from other hospitals from 1792 through 1794 are in these cartons.

3. Armées de la Moselle, carton 28, ibid.

4. Armées du Nord, carton 25, ibid.

5. Armées du Rhin, carton 29, ibid.; Jean Jomard, "Observations sur la fièvre régnant dans les hôpitaux du armée du Rhin," report to the Council of Health, 10 germinal 1793.

6. Armées du Nord, carton 25, ibid.; A. Yardin, *L'Hôpital militaire de Calais* (Paris, 1938), pp.103−5.

7. Conseil de Santé documents, carton 13, Arch. hist. Service de Santé.

8. Percy dossier, carton 211 bis, Val-de-Grâce.

9. Lafont-Gouzi dossier, carton 209, ibid.

10. Percy dossier, carton 211 bis, ibid.

11. Ibid.; Laurent, *Percy*, p.358.

12. Max Bihan, "Coste" (paper presented to the Congress of the Société Internationale d'histoire de la Médecine at Sienne, September 22−28, 1968), p.2, Coste dossier, carton 205/1, Val-de-Grâce.

13. Michel Tennetar, *Traitement de la Dyssenterie qui régne dans le département de la Moselle* (Metz, 1793), p.17.

14. Lafont-Gouzi, *Matériaux*, pp.70−71, 80.

15. Briot, *Chirurgie militaire*, pp.235−37.

16. Percy dossier, carton 211 bis, Val-de-Grâce.

17. Armées du Rhin, carton 29, Arch. hist. Service de Santé.

18. Rapports aux inspecteurs-généraux, carton 21, ibid.

19. Armées du Rhin, carton 29, ibid.

20. "Programme des cours révolutionnaires sur l'art militaire, l'administration militaire, la santé des troupes et les moyens de conserver—fait aux élèves de l'Ecole de Mars depuis le 5 fructidor jusqu'au 13 vendémiaire an III de la République" (Paris: Imprimé par ordre du Comité de Salut Public, an III), Laws and Decrees, carton 1, ibid.

21. Ibid.

22. Conseil de Santé documents, carton 13, ibid.; Rapports aux inspecteurs-généraux, carton 21, ibid.

23. Tourtelle dossier, carton 213/1, Val-de-Grâce.

24. Bretonneau dossier, carton 203, ibid.; Rapports aux inspecteurs-généraux, carton 22, Arch. hist. Service de Santé.

25. Ackernecht, *Paris hospital*, p.155.

26. Ibid., p.141.

27. Owsei Temkin, "The Role of Surgery in the Rise of Modern Medical Thought," *Bull. Hist. Med.* 25: 257.

28. Ackernecht, *Paris Hospital*, pp.47—49.

29. Corvisart dossier, carton 205/1, Val-de-Grâce.

30. Coze dossier, carton 205/1, ibid.

31. Armées du Rhin, carton 29, Arch. hist. Service de Santé.

32. Conseil de Santé documents, carton 18, ibid.

33. Guérin dossier, carton 207/3, Val-de-Grâce.

34. Armées du Rhin, carton 29, Arch. hist. Service de Santé.

35. Ibid.

36. Briot dossier, carton BII 204, Val-de-Grâce.

37. Conseil de Santé documents, cartons 11 and 12, passim, Arch. hist. Service de Santé.

38. Leclerc dossier, carton 205/1, Val-de-Grâce; Dumas dossier, carton 206/1, ibid.

39. George Rosen, *The Specialization of Medicine* (New York, 1944), p.16.

40. Temkin, "Role of Surgery," *Bull. Hist. Med.* 25: 256.

41. Ibid., 257, 259.

Chapter Nine

THE RESTORATION OF MEDICAL TRAINING

The French armies hastily mobilized by the Committee of Public Safety had checked their enemies on all fronts by late 1793, but the certainty of renewed hostilities in the spring of 1794 required a winter of feverish activity and preparation. Having pulled into its hands virtually dictatorial powers and complete jurisdiction by the Law of 14 Frimaire, the Great Committee of Public Safety was at the center of everything. Carnot, Prieur de la Côte-d'Or, and Lindet undertook to reorganize and supply the armies. The amalgamation of regular troops and the volunteers, vigorously pushed in early 1794, rebuilt the armies into coherent regiments (demi-brigades). By May 7, military command had been regularized, promotions standardized, and discipline again established through courts-martial. Nearly one million men were available for military service, and the arms industry that the Terror had organized worked frantically to provide their weapons.[1]

Military medicine was still being improvised under the supervision of the Committee of Public Safety and its representatives on mission, because the Law of August 7, 1793, had never been implemented. The terrible loss of medical officers (over 30 percent during the campaign of late 1793) had once again left the medical service with too few experienced physicians and surgeons. Out of 2,700 health officers enrolled in 1793, nearly 1,000 had been lost to wounds and disease.[2] The respite afforded by the winter months of early 1794 had to be used to secure competent replacements and to find additional health officers to serve the vast numbers of troops being readied for the coming spring campaign.

With this aim in mind, the Council of Health began circularizing all departments as early as February 9, advising them that the Council was forwarding examinations for prospective military health officers. Local authorities were to administer these tests. Candidates for commissions as health officers were to be given five hours in which to write answers to three broad medical questions. The answers were then to be sealed and returned immediately to the Council.[3] At the same time, army health officers were being given similar examinations designed to eliminate some of the incompetents already in service. The first part of the examination contained questions on amputation techniques, wounds made by firearms, and the value of mineral baths, while the second part questioned the health officer's knowledge of anatomy and pathology.[4]

Despite some absurd answers, the acute shortage of medical officers forbade the elimination of any but the worst of the incompetents, especially since the list of qualified men submitted by the departments turned out to be woefully inadequate for military needs. Even this listing proved to be unreliable, as evidenced by the commissioning of one Philibert Joseph Roux of Auxerre. His father, a military surgeon at the Auxerre hospital, answered the questions on the Council of Health's examination in order to qualify his son for a commission and, at fifteen and one-half years of age, young Roux became a surgeon third-class in the Army of the Rhine.[5]

In the midst of these examinations being conducted by the Council of Health, the Convention decided on February 24 to abolish the Council. A new organization for military medicine was created (the Law of 3 Ventôse, an II), designed to supplant the abortive law of August 7 and to put an end to the irregular operation under the representatives on mission. Control and supervision of physicians, surgeons, and pharmacists in the military medical service was to be vested in a Health Commission, supervised directly by the Provisional Executive Council. For the surveillance of "all interior details of the service," the Law of 3 Ventôse created a "police administration" composed of men employed by the Executive Council.[6]

Military hospital administration, however, was separated from any control by the Health Commission. A new Supervisory Administrative Committee was created for the direction of all military hospitals. The administration of each hospital was to be placed in the hands of a hospital committee made up of two members of the local Committee of Public Safety, two municipal officers, and a "temporary" commandant. The latter was to be temporary until his ability, efficiency, and patriotism could be investigated. All medical men and supply officers in the military hospitals were declared to be responsible to these administrative committees, who would direct all medical operations and treatments and receive regular reports from the medical staff members.[7]

In the rapidly shifting organizational decrees of early 1794, a frantic concern for the state of military medicine was evident, as well as a great deal of confusion. The new Health Commission lasted less than two weeks.

The Committee of Public Safety replaced it on March 3 with another Council of Health located in the War Ministry, composed this time of Fourcroy, Guyton de Morveau, and two others.[8] This regime was finally regularized by the Convention's decree of March 30. It approved of Carnot's proposal to suppress the Provisional Executive Council and replace the six ministries with twelve commissions.[9] Responsibility was once again centralized in a Commission of Public Assistance, which was charged with the administration of civilian hospitals, military hospitals ("both field and fixed hospitals of the armies and in the military divisions"), their personnel, materiel, cleanliness, and routine. The supervisory agents of this Commission were to check on all financial accounts, register deaths, and supervise the proper interment of the dead. To these agents was also given the responsibility for surveillance of the treatment of patients in the hospitals, in the encampments, and in the field.[10]

Despite the law of March 30, the Council of Health refused to give way to the Commission of Public Assistance on matters affecting military medicine. The struggle for control that ensued in early April threatened to wreck efforts to strengthen the medical service. Indicative of the heat involved in this quarrel was the tone of a letter from the Commission of Public Assistance to the Council of Health: "The Commission had been astonished at your inaction. You have made no response to the numerous letters which have been forwarded to you in April . . . . Do not forget that the *Revolutionary* government is involved in an extremely critical activity, that your government *is revolutionary until the peace, and that resistance to Revolutionary government is an offense against Liberty*."[11]

This deadlock forced the Convention to further action. As the spring campaign got under way, the Commission of Public Assistance was replaced by still another Council of Health. Appointed May 4–6, 1794, it was composed of the physicians Lassus, Beçu, and Paris; the surgeons Dubois, Lacoste, Berthollet, Vergez, Groffier, Chabrol, and Villar; and the pharmacists Bayen, Biron, Ducos, Hégo, Pelletier, and Théry.[12] The new importance of surgeons was reflected in the composition of the council and a clear majority of its members now had first-hand military medical experience behind them.

Meanwhile, the Committee of Public Safety decreed that the patriotism of all French health officers was to be investigated and their qualifications examined once again. The Committee of Public Safety's war commissioners were required to classify all medical men in the armies by name, age, place of birth, pay, number of campaigns, and testimonials to their patriotism. This information was to be certified by the senior medical authorities. When this was done, the war commissioners could then issue licenses and certificates of patriotism to those who were considered qualified.[13] Men serving in the regiments in nonmedical capacities could be licensed if they were able to prove one year of medical study or pass the three-question examination and successfully perform a few medical exercises (wound treatment and bandaging) under the supervision of town authorities or military medical men.[14]

The shortage of qualified physicians and surgeons, however, was simply not to be remedied by these measures. As the spring campaign opened badly for France, with Landrécies surrendering on April 30 and Cambrai threatened, the increasingly pressing need for any sort of health officer led to some extraordinarily easy evaluations of competence. For example, an old farm worker named Charaux was commissioned as a pharmacist because he had "in his youth been apprenticed in pharmacy."[15] By the summer of 1794, the number of health officers had been raised to four thousand but incompetence was still tolerated and the military medical service was still handled as before on an emergency basis.[16]

The Committee of Public Safety was slowly turning to thoughts of reviving medical education. In February, 1794, it had successfully launched a technical school, the Ecole des armes, to meet the acute shortage of skilled manpower and to help manufacture the arms needed for victory. The National School of Roads and Bridges was reorganized to provide the nation with desperately needed engineers. Formal military training, which had been crippled by the Convention in September of 1793, was resumed under plans formulated in May of 1794, and the Ecole de Mars was in operation by late June.[17] Since March, various plans had been under study for the resumption of formal medical training. From the ambulance hospitals at Mayence, Briot had proposed simply increasing the number of corpsmen and students, setting up first-aid camps near the armies in the field, and letting the students help and learn while actually treating the wounded.[18] A proposal by Maurice and Fages called for the creation of special teaching hospitals similar to the prerevolutionary amphitheaters.[19] A plan by Noël, Gilbert, and Brougniart of Val-de-Grâce advocated a process for selecting students 15 to 18 years of age and putting them in the nearest military hospital for training as physicians, surgeons, or pharmacists.[20] The spring and early summer of 1794 brought no agreement as to which plan should be implemented. The basic disagreement lay between the idea of several big teaching hospitals (considered by some only as disguised medical schools) and the use of military hospitals as teaching centers.

Finally, on July 13, the Committee of Public Safety decided to reinstate formal medical education. It decreed the establishment of a "revolutionary school of the art of healing" and named Antoine Fourcroy and François Chaussier to draw up plans for the new school. Chaussier, an anatomist from Dijon whose treatise on legal medicine (1790) heralded the advent of a new medical specialty in France, assumed the main burden of preparing the proposal. The Committee authorized Chaussier to be paid at the rate of 600 livres per month while he was in Paris working on this project.[21]

However, Chaussier's work was frequently interrupted. The events of 9 Thermidor, which brought down Robespierre and eventually ended the Terror, delayed his concentration on the proposed "School of Health" for almost a month. In September, the new Committee of Public Safety required Chaussier to prepare and deliver lectures at the Ecole de Mars on personal hygiene and on contagious and epidemic diseases. Then the death of the celebrated comparative anatomist, Félix Vicq d'Azyr, required that someone of Chaussier's stature purchase Vicq's manuscripts and instruments, catalogue and preserve them, and continue his experiments, so the Commitee of Public Safety ordered Chaussier to this task on September 22, 1794.[22]

The strain on Chaussier was eased somewhat by the expert assistants assigned to him: the technical artist Pierre Joseph Redoute (1759–1840), famed for the detail and exactness of his drawings and plates, and Jean Baptiste Huzard (1755–1838), a veterinarian and agriculturist who had collaborated with Vicq and was familiar with his research.[23] Six commissioners, with Fourcroy as chairman, were also designated to assist Chaussier in perfecting plans for renewing medical education. Thuriot, Treilhard, and C. A. Prieur were drawn from the Committee of Public Safety and the physicians Duhem, Plaichard, and Fourcroy represented the Committee of Public Education. Under the arrangement that developed, Chaussier was left to propose the curriculum while Fourcroy turned his attention to problems of organization and administration.[24] The fall of 1794 was devoted to efforts to formulate a plan for restoring formal medical education in France that could win acceptance by the Convention.

In the meantime, the Committee of Public Safety was kept vividly aware of the dwindling ranks of military medical men by the ferocity of epidemic illnesses left in the wake of the armies and from time to time it issued decrees to aid in combatting them. One physician, Dufau of Mont-de-Marsan, convinced the Committee that these epidemics were not climatic or hereditary diseases. He asserted, "A multitude of facts show that the itch, venereal diseases, etc. pass from infected subjects to healthy subjects, by more or less immediate contact or by sexual intercourse."[25] Therefore the Committee took drastic action on August 24, 1794, prohibiting any soldier from using a barracks bed if he had the itch or any other communicable disease. A bed occupied by such a person or commandeered for use in a hospital or quarantine area was not to be used in a barracks again. All of the beds of this nature were to be retained for hospital use and the word "hospital" was to be burned into the wooden bedstead. All sheets and mattresses used by any person with a communicable disease were to be similarly marked and anyone caught altering any of these required markings was to be imprisoned for a month.[26]

As the fortunes of war again shifted to favor France in the summer of 1794, the fierce fighting produced heavy casualties. General Jourdan took Charleroi at about the same time General Pichegru seized Ypres. The victory at Fleurus on June 26 opened the way to Belgium where Jourdan and Pichegru soon joined forces in Brussels. Liège fell, and Antwerp surrendered to the French armies on July 27. The military medical service could not cope with the results of engagements such as the one at Aywaille on September 18. The French approached a narrow bridge defended by Austrian twelve-pounders firing case-shot at point-blank range. To the consternation of health officers, the dead and wounded who obstructed passage over the bridge were thrown into the river as the French troops forced their way across.[27] The carnage at Aywaille rather than being an isolated occurrence was characteristic of the fall campaign of 1794.

Few perished in combat, however, compared to the sick and wounded who were left strewn in the wake of the advancing French armies. The Austrians left their wounded behind to be tended by French military medical men. At Liège alone, 6,500 wounded jammed the hospitals which had been stripped of equipment and furnishings by the retreating Austrians. In an area where the itch was endemic, the vast numbers of men passing through raised it soon to epidemic proportions. The straw upon which the majority of the wounded lay provided a perfect means of spreading all contagious diseases.[28] General Pichegru himself came down with the itch in September and requested a leave in order to recover. On October 10, Lacombe reported to the Committee of Public Safety from Ryswick that both the armies of the Sambre-et-Meuse and the North were overwhelmed by the itch, and the next day, Bellegarde wrote that Pichegru had been ill with it for nearly a month.[29]

From the Vendée, Boursault reported at the same time (October 10) that such a widespread epidemic of itch (*gale*) existed that "these *galériens* have become the most dangerous agents" of the rebels.[30] In the Army of the Maritime Alps, an epidemic marked by diarrhea, colic, and high fever struck and virtually paralyzed the Italian front. Of a concentration of 24,000 troops on the Genes River, 16,000 were sick, and further north, Kellermann's army of 87,500 had only an estimated 44,000 fit for duty.[31] Delbrel had written to the Committee of Public Safety that the Army of the Eastern Pyrenees had 30,000 sick on September 30, and by October 12 he was terming the number affected by the epidemic as "shocking." Their condition was the more critical because the hospitals could not begin to cope with such staggering aggregations of sick men. Yet they could not be sent home, Delbrel said, "because they cannot get food on their journey."[32] Besides, many were afflicted with anthrax, or local carbuncle, and could not walk at all.[33]

In desperation, the Committee of Public Safety issued a decree permitting the sick and wounded to be nursed at home. Profiting from earlier mistakes along this line, however, the Committee's order notified municipal authorities that they would be responsible and held strictly accountable for seeing that troops returning home stayed only until they were well again.[34] Various epidemic areas were furnished with teams of medical men drafted by the Committee of Public Safety to try to control the spread of disease as quickly as possible.[35] To provide for the hordes suffering with the itch, mineral springs and baths were recommended by the Committee. Agents were dispatched to open up many of the mineral spring resorts which had formerly been used by the wealthy. On October 17, the Committee ordered wide publicity given to the healing qualities of these resorts and authorized the publication of 5,000 copies of Antoine Lomet's pamphlet, *Mémoire sur les eaux minérales et les etablissements thermaux des Pyrénées*.[36] This widely distributed pamphlet also permitted the authorities of any area where warm springs were available to construct their own health baths. By following Lomet's descriptions and instructions, hundreds of these mineral baths were created by local workmen in response to the Committee of Public Safety's appeal for immediate facilities for "curing the wounds of the defenders of the Republic and for alleviating the suffering of humanity."[37]

A renewed virulence of venereal disease in the armies moving into Spain, Belgium, and the Palatinate in the fall of 1794 could not be controlled by the Committee of Public Safety's decrees that sought to "fix the number of women who could accompany soldiers to bed or battle."[38] The acute shortage of mercury, the standard treatment, encouraged the Committee to test the claims of Jean Stanislaus Mittie who had been trying since 1789 to convince the French medical profession of the value of his plan "to cure all [venereal] diseases" with "vegetables alone."[39] Mittie was given a provincial hospital and assigned a team of physicians, surgeons, and apothecaries. This team was to prepare all medicines, administer them, and make regular progress reports to the Committee of Public Safety. Twenty soldiers were assigned to Mittie's hospital, chosen on the basis of their varied stages of venereal infection. Mittie prohibited the use of any preparation containing mercury or any other mineral in treating his patients, but the whole experiment was a dismal failure. By December of 1794, the Committee of Public Safety was once again trying vigorously to increase the production of mercury, in order to deal with the steadily mounting incidence of venereal infection in the armies.[40]

To combat the shortage of medicines and medical equipment, the Committee of Public Safety ordered Guillaume Daignan to new duties on October 22. First on the Council of Health, then released to do research on nutrition, Daignan was given the task of collecting medicines and preparing the bottles for shipment to the armies and military hospitals.[41] Legros, an orthopedist, was put to work making artificial limbs, and Laumonier, the chief health officer at the hospital in Rouen, was ordered to produce teaching aids in anticipation of the renewal of medical education in the Ecole de Santé that Chaussier was planning. The Committee of Public Safety ordered an artificial anatomy which could be assembled and disassembled to reveal the whole lymphatic system and another to reveal the nervous system. Laumonier was given 500 pounds of mercury to assist him in tracing out the fine outlines of both systems, and a stipend of 5,000 livres.[42]

To ease the lot of the struggling medical service, the Committee of Public Safety returned to active duty a great many of the physicians and surgeons who had been suspended for disloyalty by representatives on mission since September 12, 1791.[43] Captured physicians and surgeons were sent to the interior hospitals to treat the sick and wounded, and at times were permitted to engage in private practice in the communities in which the hospitals were located. The new uniforms that were being issued to health officers were resplendent with brass buttons, engraved around the edges with the words *"Hôpitaux militaires"* and in the center, *"Humanité."* The Committee of Public Safety also granted to all health officers attached to the military hospitals exemption from standing guard duty, provided they paid someone to mount guard for them.[44]

Finally, the Committee of Public Safety conceded on December 26 that the Law of 3 Ventôse which regulated the military medical service was simply unenforceable. The shortage of medical men was too acute to attempt to follow rigid rules about the capacity, training, and zeal of the men commissioned as health officers. Rather lamely, therefore, the Committee thought that the best procedure was to ask the chief medical officers of the armies and of the military hospitals to "assure themselves as to the capacity of their collaborators." At the same time, French conquests in the Low Countries prompted the reorganization of the Army of the North. Hospitals in the "Military Zone of the Exterior" were distinguished from hospitals in the interior of France. Military medical supervision was confirmed in hospitals in Flanders, Belgium, Brabant, and Holland. Outside of France, hospitals would be supplied by requisitioning among the conquered people. The interior hospitals, in the departments of Nord, Pas-de-Calais, Oise, Somme, Aisne, and Seine-et-Marne passed under the control of the Committee of Public Welfare.[45]

Although Chaussier continued to labor through 1794 on a detailed plan for medical and surgical training, France's agonizing need for competent health officers for the armies led the committee of six commissioners to present a plan to the National Convention on November 27. As chairman, Fourcroy read the report and the proposed decree. The plan that was suggested for the Central School of Health for training physicians and surgeons was the same as that of the Ecole de Mars and the Ecole centrale des travaux publics. It was to be one great national medical institution, which would draw outstanding students to Paris from all parts of the country. The course of study was to cover three years, and the students were to be classified into three groups. This was little more than a revival of the practice that had been common in military medical amphitheaters under the Old Regime. The commençants could anticipate three full years of study. Commencés, or students with some medical study or experience, could graduate sooner, while the avancés were those considered by the faculty to be capable of graduation in one year or less.[46]

During the debate, which lasted from November 27 to December 4, 1794, only two major reactions emerged. One was the strong feeling that it was urgent to produce medical officers for the armies. The plan for classifying students as avancés who could be graduated quickly was appealing in an atmosphere that reflected an elaborate concern for the sick and wounded defenders of the nation. One Convention spokesman, Rochard, summarized his support by saying impatiently, "Practice them [the avancés] in operations and send them to complete their apprenticeship on the field of battle."[47]

The other reaction in the Convention was negative. Sectional feeling objected strenuously to a single great School of Health located in Paris. Deputies from southern France advanced the claims of the great medical facility at Montpellier. Many others cited Strasbourg, a center of military medical training for almost a century, as a logical site. The result was that the Convention became adamant on one point: there would be no one great medical school located at Paris. In debate, a compromise was hammered out. The proposed 550 medical students would be divided up among three schools: 300 at Paris, 150 at Montpellier, and 100 at Strasbourg.[48] Having satisfied regional interests and successfully preserved two old and honorable centers of medical training, the Convention speedily approved the modified proposal on December 4, 1794.

This Law of 14 Frimaire announced that the three medical schools would be especially designed to produce health officers for military and naval service. It assigned to the Strasbourg school the same amphitheater building that had been used as a school of military medicine and surgery under the Old Regime. The Montpellier school was to have the same facilities that the University of Montpellier had traditionally used for medical teaching. In Paris, the magnificent building that had formerly housed the Academy of Surgery would accommodate the Paris School of Health, although the former convent of the Cordeliers was later added to these facilities in view of the 300 students who were to be enrolled. Article VIII of the Law of 14 Frimaire took care of any legal complications by declaring the defunct schools of surgery at Paris, Montpellier, and Strasbourg to be "suppressed" and, at the same time, "merged with the new Schools of Health which are established by this decree."[49]

Each school was to have a library (though only Paris would have a librarian), an anatomy laboratory, a cabinet of surgical instruments and equipment, and a collection of items of natural history. The Committee of Public Safety turned over to the Committee of Public Education the task of gathering up from the various national depots the necessary equipment and materials for each school. They would be delivered through the school director to a custodian who would be responsible for all property of the school. Six professors were authorized for Strasbourg, eight for Montpellier, and twelve for the Paris school. They would be appointed by the Committee of Public Education and each professor would be given an assistant "so that the lessons and other responsibilities relative to the teaching and perfecting of the art of healing shall never be interrupted."[50]

Each district of the Republic was to furnish a student who was between the ages of 17 and 26 years. This student would be chosen by a committee composed of two health officers in the district capital (named by the Commission of Health) and one citizen "notable for his republican virtues" (named by the District Directory). This committee was required to select on the basis of the candidate's "patriotism and upon his background of knowledge acquired in one or more of the sciences basic to the art of healing, such as anatomy, chemistry, natural history, or physics."[51] The chosen student would be given "nomination papers" signed by the selection committee and by the district's national agent. He was to be instructed to go to the nearest School of Health and received pay for his trip at the rate of an artilleryman first class. The student was expected to arrive at his destination by January 19, 1795, the day the medical schools were set to open.[52]

Upon arrival at Paris, Montpellier, or Strasbourg, the medical students would be classified as commençants, commencés, or avancés, according to their nomination papers. The decree made clear the urgent priority being assigned to military medical service by emphasizing that "those who, *at whatever point in their studies*, have acquired the necessary knowledge to practice the art of healing in the hospitals and in the armies, will be used in that service by the Commission of Health," when the latter was informed of this by the student's professors.[53] Such students, leaving before a full three years of study, were to be replaced immediately by other qualified students chosen from the districts of the students leaving the medical schools. While in school, the students were to be paid at the same rate as those in the Ecole centrale des travaux publics, but the decree left the salaries of professors, assistant professors, directors, custodians, and other employees to be set by agreement between the Committee of Public Education and the Committee of Finance.[54]

The curriculum to be followed in the medical schools included "the structure and physics of man, the symptoms and characteristics of illnesses . . . the known means of cure, and properties of plants and of ordinary drugs, medical chemistry, the techniques of operations, the use of instruments, the application of bandages, and the public duties of health officers."[55] In addition, medical students would observe the treatment of patients, watch surgical operations, and later serve as interns in local hospitals near their schools. The general wording of this part of the Law of 14 Frimaire reflected the fact that Chaussier's work had been incomplete when Fourcroy's committee had been required to report to the Convention. The vague wording of this Article III ultimately proved to be fortunate, however, because it could be construed later to include new courses which incorporated the knowledge gained from the military campaigns since 1792. Having at last authorized the reinstitution of medical and surgical training that had been suppressed in France since 1790, the Convention gave its supervision to the Committee of Public Education and required it to "take all necessary measures to insure the execution" of its decree of December 4, 1794.[56]

The year that had begun with frantic efforts to secure military health officers and with the rapidly shifting organizational changes of February 24, March 3, March 30, and April 17, ended with a fairly definitive plan for regular medical education. The Committee of Public Safety had followed expedients only until the Republic was no longer in peril and then, on the basis of its successful Ecole de Mars and Ecole centrale des travaux publics, it sought to create stable and productive medical schools. The great urgency of the Committee of Public Safety's interest in this stemmed from the visibly thinning ranks of experienced military medical men, the extraordinarily widespread incidence of epidemic diseases in 1794, and the Committee's conclusion that no effective and enforceable decree on the organization of military medicine was possible without trained medical personnel.

Whatever its motives, the Convention had adopted some new principles of medicine and medical education which now became fundamentals of the "new medicine." The following sections, in Fourcroy's report to the Convention on November 27, 1794, were of tremendous significance for the future of French medicine: "It is not sufficient to give lessons and public courses on all branches of science. The old method did not give a complete course and was limited to words .... Once the lesson was finished, its contents vanished from the students' memory. In the Ecole de Santé practice will be united with theoretical precepts. The students will do chemical experiments, dissections, operations and bandaging. Little reading, much seeing, and much doing will be the foundation of the new teaching which your Committee suggests. Practicing the art [of healing], observing at the bedside, all that was missing, will now be the principal part of instruction .... Your intention to revive useful science and to further its progress makes it necessary that the professors and their associates have only this function and are not distracted by other occupations. Therefore, their salaries must be sufficient for their needs, and they must not be obliged to do additional work in order to subsist .... Medicine and surgery are two branches of the same science. To study them separately means to abandon theory to delirious imagination and practice to blind routine. To reunite them and to melt them together means to enlighten them mutually and to further their progress .... "[57]

Four great principles of the new medicine were clearly defined in Fourcroy's report, which served as the basis of the Law of 14 Frimaire, an III (December 4, 1794) for the resumption of formal medical education. First, there was a vindication of prerevolutionary clinical teaching and a solid endorsement of the practical medical instruction of the war years.

The new theory of medical education emphasized the clinical approach that had been advocated by Cabanis, Desault, Pinel, and Corvisart. Students at the new medical schools would begin their studies not with theoretical instruction but with the practical experience to be derived from actually doing "chemical experiments, dissections, operations and bandaging,"[58] depending upon whatever previous experience they brought with them. The preponderance of anatomy and pathology and the immediacy of applied instruction was to be insured by practical training in dissection, an approach guaranteed by the authorization of five hundred cadavers for each school in its first year.

A second principle of paramount importance was the unquestioned acceptance of the hospital as the appropriate training ground for physicians and surgeons. From his first day in medical school, the new student would be put into the hospital wards. This was the way really to become a medical practitioner and to acquire the ability to observe the signs of illness and disease accurately and scientifically. As Fourcroy said, "practicing the art, observing at the bedside . . . little reading, much seeing and much doing will be the foundation of the new teaching."[59] And it was the hospital that was now the accepted institution for such instruction, so much so that instruction by the Paris faculty was described as "hospital staffs engaged in teaching."[60]

The third significant principle was Fourcroy's emphasis upon full-time professors, financially emancipated from their students and able, ideally, to devote themselves exclusively to their teaching roles. While this ideal was not entirely met, the chairs established in the new medical schools carried with them stipends sufficiently generous to insure stiff competition from among the ablest medical teachers in France. The practice of *permutation* allowed a professor priority in obtaining a more attractive chair when it became vacant within his school. Also, there was no prohibition against holding teaching positions simultaneously, in the Ecole de Santé and in a private lycée (Fourcroy himself held three chairs at one time in three different schools).[61] Nor was private practice ruled out. Consequently, in striking contrast with the old prerevolutionary faculty who refused to practice what they taught, the new faculty was actively engaged in private practice.

Finally, the fourth principle laid down in Fourcroy's report was the reunification of medicine and surgery. While the antecedents of this development had been visible before the Revolution, the events of 1789 and of the war years following had accelerated its progress and had, in fact, effected the reunion. As Ackernecht has aptly put it, "This was indeed an event of great historical and international importance. It was the closing hour of medical medievalism."[62] Stated another way, the law that authorized the reinstitution of medical education in 1795 left no doubt that medicine and surgery had been reunited and that a new era was dawning in French medicine.

NOTES

1. Lefebvre, *French Revolution from 1793 to 1799*, pp.92–98; Palmer, *Twelve Who Ruled*, p.127.

2. Departments, carton 4, Arch. hist. Service de Santé; Rieux and Hassenforder, *Histoire*, p.20; Cilleuls, "Les médecins aux armées," *Revue hist. de l'armée* 6: 24.

3. Conseil de Santé documents, carton 12, Arch. hist. Service de Santé. Cochin and Charpentier, *Les actes* 2: 267–68. Members of the Council of Health were Heurteloup, A. Dubois, Bassi, Bayen, Hégot, Parmentier, and Théry.

4. Percy dossier, carton 211 bis, Val-de-Grâce; Laurent, *Percy*, pp.146–52.

5. Conseil de Santé documents, carton 10, Arch. hist. Service de Santé. Apparently this sort of fraud was common. When Roux's incapacity was discovered, nothing was done about it.

6. Conseil de Santé documents, carton 18, ibid. The text of this hastily drafted and ill-conceived legislation is also in *Dict. encyclopédique sci. méd.*, 2d ser., 8: 96–97.

7. Conseil de Santé documents, carton 13, Arch. hist. Service de Santé.

8. Conseil de Santé documents, carton 18, ibid.; Smeaton, *Fourcroy*, p.62.

9. Guillaume, *Convention* 4: 67–68.

10. Ganges, *Représentants du peuple* 1: 437–39.

11. Conseil de Santé correspondence, carton 20, Arch. hist. Service de Santé. Italics in the original letter, dated May 2, 1794.

12. Rapports aux inspecteurs-généraux, carton 21, ibid.

13. Cochin and Charpentier, *Les actes* 3: 109–10.

14. Conseil de Santé documents, carton 18, Arch. hist. Service de Santé; Cabanès, *Chirurgiens et blessés*, p.339.

15. Aulard, *Recueil des actes* 19: 729.

16. Rieux and Hassenforder, *Histoire*, p.20.

17. *Moniteur* 16: 662ff.; 17: 608; 20: 622–27.

18. Armées du Rhin, carton 29, Arch. hist. Service de Santé; original handwritten proposal by Briot.

19. Conseil de Santé documents, carton 13, ibid.; original proposal entitled, "Observations et projets de J. B. Maurice et Fages sur la création des Hôpitaux d'Instruction (29 mars 1794)."

20. The original of this plan is in carton 20, ibid.

21. Aulard, *Recueil des actes* 15: 132. François Chaussier of Dijon (1746–1828), a modest and conscientious physician and a prolific writer. He pioneered the study of law as it related to the medical profession. Legal cases involving accidents, damage claims, liability, and negligence were brought together into a comprehensive study for the first time in France. When medical training was resumed in 1794, this infant field of legal medicine was included in the curriculum. Its greatest value at that time lay in the emphasis that could be placed upon injuries arising out of accidents. A loosely defined area, legal medicine courses served to permit teaching the new concepts of wounds and wound treatments derived from wartime experiences while the medical schools simultaneously honored the Convention's demand that the older Hippocratic methods be taught. See *Nouvelle biographie*, 10: 147–49.

22. Aulard, *Recueil des actes* 17: 20, 85; 20: 453–54; Guillaume, *Convention* 5: xl, 81–82.

23. Aulard, *Recueil des actes* 17: 20–21.

24. Guillaume, *Convention* 4: xxxiii. This joint committee worked primarily on organization and left to Chaussier the problems of curriculum.

25. Cabanès, *Chirurgiens et blessés*, p.333.

26. Conseil de Santé documents, carton 13, Arch. hist. Service de Santé; Aulard, *Recueil des actes* 16: 69–70.

27. Phipps, *Armies of the First Republic* 2: 182.

28. Ganges, *Représentants du peuple* 3: 107–8.

29. Aulard, *Recueil des actes* 17: 6, 346, 367.

30. Ibid., 17: 348.

31. Larrey, *Memoirs* 1: 40–41; Ganges, *Représentants du peuple* 3: 108–9.

32. Aulard, *Recueil des actes* 17: 163, 396.

33. Larrey, *Memoirs* 1: 52–54.

34. Cochin and Charpentier, *Les actes* 3: 524–25.

35. Aulard, *Recueil des actes* 12: 753; 16: 720–21; 17: 672; 18: 544; 20: 542.

36. Ibid., 10: 373; 17: 478. Antoine François Lomet (1759–1826), an engineer and graduate of the School of Roads and Bridges. See *Nouvelle biographie* 31: 537–38.

37. Aulard, *Recueil des actes* 18: 275.

38. Brooks Thompson, "The Wartime Mobilization of Savants by the Committees of Public Safety" (doctoral dissertation, University of Alabama, 1955), p.285.

39. *Arch. Parl.*, 74: 567, 607—16. Jean Stanislaus Mittie (1727—95), one-time member of the Faculty of Medicine of Paris and former physician to Stanislaus Lesczynski of Poland and Lorraine.

40. Aulard, *Recueil des actes* 20: 242; 21: 373,424.

41. Ibid., 17: 559.

42. Guillaume, *Convention* 5: 589.

43. *Loi relatif aux officiers privés de leur état sans cause légitime or arbitrarement suspendus de leur fonctions depuis 12 septembre 1791* (Paris: Imprimerie Nationale executive du Louvre, 1793), Laws and Decrees, carton 1, Arch. hist. Service de Santé.

44. Aulard, *Recueil des actes* 19: 187—89; Cabanès, *Chirurgiens et blessés*, p.352.

45. Aulard, *Recueil des actes* 19: 101—2.

46. *Moniteur* 22: 618, 663—67, 721; Guillaume, *Convention* 4: xxxiii, 980; Smeaton, *Fourcroy*, p.62.

47. Quoted in Laignel-Lavastine, *Histoire générale* 2: 449. See Cabanès, *Chirurgiens et blessés* pp.334—51, for an account of the somewhat exaggerated honors and special holidays devoted to recognition of the wounded.

48. *Moniteur* 22: 721: Guillaume, *Convention* 4: xxxiv, 980.

49. See Articles I, II, and VIII in Guillaume, *Convention* 5: 281—82.

50. Ibid. See Articles V and VI.

51. Ibid. See Articles IX and X.

52. Ibid., 4: 980; 5: 282. See Articles VII and XI.

53. Ibid. Italics mine. See Article XII.

54. Ibid. See Articles XIII and XIV.

55. Ibid. See Articles III and IV.

56. Ibid., 5: 283.

57. Ibid., 4: 980; *Moniteur* 22: 663—67.

58. Ibid.

59. Ibid.

60. Ackernecht, *Paris Hospital* p.37, quoting Abraham Flexner.

61. Ibid., p.33.

62. Ibid.

Chapter Ten

THE THERMIDORIANS
AND FRENCH MEDICINE

The Committee of Public Education, headed by Fourcroy, was charged by the Law of December 4, 1794, with responsibility for reinstituting medical training in France. The physicians René Plaichard and Jean Barailon were designated to assist Fourcroy in carrying out the National Convention's decree, and these three now constituted a new Commission of Health.[1] Copies of the new law were rushed to all agents of the Committee of Public Safety, while the Commission of Health marked out the 550 districts of France from which the medical students were to be drawn. At the same time, the commission began the slow job of preparing a list of provincial health officers who could serve as examiners of candidates for the new medical schools. However, an appalling lack of information and the general scarcity of health officers made this task almost impossible to accomplish in Paris. It was a job rendered all the more difficult because of the somewhat hysterical pressure from other members of the Committee of Public Education, who kept urging Fourcroy, Plaichard, and Barailon to hurry the nomination of examiners.[2] The prospective examiners, on the other hand, had by law been given fifteen days in which to submit affidavits concerning their personal lives, titles, and length of study.[3]

In desperation, the Committee of Public Safety intervened on December 20 with a formal decree. Article I of the decree gave the Commission of Health just two days in which to submit a list of district health officers who were to examine and nominate candidates to the medical schools. Article II, however, urged the submission of an incomplete list in view of the urgency of getting medical education underway. The Commission of Health was ordered to notify immediately the representatives on mission in every district where no examiners had been located, so that these representatives could find some health officers to perform this function. The Committee of Public Safety instructed further that if enough health officers could not be found in the district capitals, the representatives were to scour the whole district for them.[4] Thus a frantic search was set in motion in nearly all of the districts for the necessary medical men to act as examiners of potential medical students.

In the same decree of December 20, the Committee of Public Safety took over the search for qualified students. Examiners were told to nominate anyone between the ages of 18 and 26 years who had one year of medical experience. This had been expressly forbidden by the Law of December 4. In order to prevent the selection of health officers serving in the armies and in military hospitals, the Committee decreed that no one could leave the medical service without a recommendation from the Commission of Health, approved by the Committee of Public Safety. Having thus frozen military health officers in their positions, the Committee then authorized the examiners in the districts where no eligible students could be found to select anyone "with some preliminary studies and an evident aptitude for instruction."[5]

The shortage of qualified students was more acute than the Committee of Public Safety even dreamed. Barailon was forced by December 29 to go before the Convention and ask for a liberalization of the Law of December 4. He spoke of the "urgent needs" of the armies for health officers and appealed for immediate changes in the law. The Convention acted at once to drop the requirement of competitive examinations. In addition, the law was broadened to permit the selection of students between the ages of 16 and 30 years. An original prohibition against the selection of men who had served as army health officers in the first draft of 1792–93 was dropped, and the Convention agreed to allow the selection of anyone, even if he were in the military service.[6] With this liberalization of the law on December 29, the Convention opened the door to formal medical training for hundreds of young military health officers who could be graduated in less than three years, many in less than one year.

While the frantic search for medical examiners and for qualified students for the medical schools proceeded, the Committee of Public Safety pushed the staffing of the new schools which were slated to open on January 19, 1795.[7] The faculty of the Paris School of Health was nominated by the Committee of Public Education on December 14:[8]

Professors	Subjects	Assistants
Hallé	Medical physics and hygiene	Pinel
Chaussier	Anatomy and physiology	Dubois
Chopart	Surgical pathology	Percy
Doublet	Medical pathology	Bourdier
Peyrilhe	Botany and medical materials	Richard

Fourcroy	Medical chemistry and pharmacy	Deyeux
Sabatier	Operative surgery	Boyer
Corvisart	Clinical medicine	Leclerc
Desault	Clinical surgery	Manoury[9]
Pelletan	Rare medical and surgical cases	Lallement
Lassus	Legal medicine	Mahon
A. LeRoy	Obstetrics	Baudelocque

On December 16, the School of Health at Montepellier was assigned its faculty:[10]

Professors	Subjects	Assistants
René	Legal medicine	
Dumas	Anatomy, physiology, applied medicine	Lafabrie
Gouan	Botany and medical materials	Amoreaux
Chaptal	Chemistry (medical, animal, and applied)	Bérard
Baumes	Pathology, drugs, and meteorology	Senaux
Montabret[11]	Operative surgery and rare cases	Broussonnet
Souquet	Clinical observation	Petiot
Poutingon	Clinical surgery	Vigarous
Laborie	Maternity, obstetrics, pediatrics	Méjean
Verinque	Librarian and records	

The School of Health at Strasbourg was not organized until December 22. The faculty recommended by the Committee of Public Education included:

Professors	Subjects	Assistants
Lauth	Anatomy, physiology, applied physics, and meteorology	Bérot
Hermann	Botany, medical materials, and natural history	Gorcy
Tourtelle	Hygiene, pathology, prophylaxis	Busch
Coze	Internal medicine	Roederer
Flamant	Theoretical and practical surgery gynecology, and pediatrics	Barbier
Nicolas	Chemistry (medical, animal, applied) and pharmacy	Hecht
Lorentz, Jr.	Legal medicine and rare cases (both medical and surgical)	
Pfeffinger[12]	Curator	

An analysis of the faculties of the three schools of health affords an insight into the new medical world that was emerging in France by early 1795. One aspect that was new was the office of a permanent dean. At Paris, this post went to Michel Auguste Thouret, who held it until his death in 1810. His teaching was confined to lectures on Hippocrates and rare cases. As dean, Thouret collaborated with Fourcroy in the selection of the Paris staff. A former member of the Royal Society of Medicine and of the National Assembly, Thouret was a friend of Cabanis and Fourcroy and a leading exponent of smallpox vaccination. His greatest talents, however, seemed to lie in medical administration. The vigorous manner in which Thouret took very disparate elements and welded them together into a new school was a testimony both to his ability and to the growing tendency toward centralized administration.[13]

To teach at Paris, some great prerevolutionary figures were selected to be professors. Jean Noël Hallé, who had been so devoted to the old Faculty of Medicine at Paris that he had refused to join the Royal Society of Medicine, became professor of medical physics.[14] Philippe Pelletan, who was named to teach rare cases, had been at the Hôtel-Dieu since his student days as an assistant to Desault.[15] The latter, who had lived through the revolutionary storm as surgeon in chief at the Hôtel-Dieu, became professor of clinical surgery. Corvisart, Desault's student who had been physician in chief at the Charité since 1788 and famous as a remarkable diagnostician, was selected to teach clinical medicine. François Chopart, noted for the foot amputation technique he had devised and a good friend and associate of Desault at the Hôtel-Dieu, was nominated to teach surgical pathology.[16] Bernard Peyrilhe, a 1769 graduate of the College of Surgery in Paris and a former member of the Royal Academy of Surgery, became professor of botany and medical materials.[17] A former surgeon to Louis XV's daughters and at one time suspect because of his lukewarm attitude toward the Revolution, Pierre Lassus was chosen to teach legal medicine.[18] The only professor with any military service was Sabatier, who was taken from his established place at the Invalides and made professor of operative surgery.[19] Selected to teach medical pathology, François Doublet had succeeded Fourcroy in 1793 as director of the Society of Medicine.[20] Chaussier, whose *Traité complet de médecine légale* (1790) was to be the text for the courses to be taught by Lassus, was appointed to teach anatomy and physiology.[21] Fourcroy (who was named to teach chemistry), Chaussier, and Doublet were the only active Jacobins who moved into top positions in the Paris school.[22]

Seven of the ten assistants at Paris came directly from military medicine. Two army surgeons, Claude Leclerc and Claude Pinson, were brought in to assist Desault and Corvisart. A military physician at the military hospital at Pont-Sainte-Maxence (Oise) named Bourdier was selected to assist Doublet in pathology.[23] Paul Mahon had been physician in chief of the Hôpital des Vénériens prior to serving with the Army of the Côtes de Cherbourg.[24] Antoine Dubois returned to Paris from the Army of the Alps, and Alexis Boyer from the Army of the North.[25] The best known assistant with military service was Percy, who left his place as surgeon in chief of the Army of the Sambre-et-Meuse.[26] Only Louis Richard, M. P. Lallement, and Phillipe Pinel had had no military medical experience. Richard was a botanist who was cool toward the Revolution and who served on the Committee of Public Safety after 9 Thermidor. Lallement had vegetated during the Revolution as surgeon in chief at the Salpêtrière. Pinel, after his famous report to the Convention in 1791 on the treatment of the insane, became chief physician at the Bicêtre. He had been denounced and arrested during the Terror but was freed after 9 Thermidor.[27] Four of these ten assistants, Boyer, Dubois, Lallement, and Mahon, were former students of Desault.[28]

The old faculty of medicine was virtually restored in the School of Health at Montpellier. Of the ten top men, nine had taught there prior to 1789: the disputatious Chaptal, the director René, Montabret (soon replaced by Broussonnet), Baumes, Laborie, Poutingon, Souquet, Gouan, and Verinque.[29] Chaptal had been a Girondin who fled to Paris when threatened with arrest and had worked during the Terror with Berthollet and Monge.[30] Antoine Gouan had been a professor at Montpellier since 1769, though he also served as a physician in the local military hospital from 1792 to 1815.[31] Only Victor Broussonnet and Charles Louis Dumas were new professors. Sabatier's student, Dumas, had succeeded Barthélemy Vigarous at Montpellier in 1791. He served with Army of Italy at Nice with Larrey in 1793 and in the Army of the Alps in 1794. Broussonnet and Dumas were the only professors who brought experience in battle surgery to the new Montpellier school.[32]

The eight assistants at Montpellier were equally home grown. Only three had military medical experience: René Bertin (who succeeded Broussonnet), Vigarous, and Lafabrie. Bertin had been with the Army of the Côtes de Brest while the latter two had served in the Army of the Eastern Pyrenees since 1792. Vigarous was the son of the former Montpellier professor of surgery, Barthélemy Vigarous.[33] The other five assistants were probably former Montpellier teachers. Méjean, Petiot, and Senaux left no mark at all on French medicine. Pierre Amoreaux was the former Montpellier librarian, and Pierre Bérard was noted chiefly as the father of two distinguished graduates of Montpellier, Auguste (b. 1802) and Pierre Honoré (b. 1797).[34]

The complexion of the faculty appointed to the School of Health at Strasbourg was quite different from that at Montpellier. Experienced military medical men were given charge of the Strasbourg school. The director, Joseph Adam Lorentz, Jr., had served in the Army of the Rhine under his famous father, who was physician in chief of that army.[35] Thomas Lauth had studied under Desault and Hunter and was physician in chief of the Strasbourg military hospital.[36] Etienne Tourtelle had served in the Army of the Rhine as a physician from 1792, as had Pierre Nicolas.[37] Pierre Coze had been surgeon-major of a royal cavalry regiment, physician in the Army of the Alps in 1792, served at the military hospital at Lyon in 1793, and at the military hospital at Metz in 1794.[38] A student of Desault, Pierre Flamant had been a professor of surgery in the military medical amphitheater in Strasbourg.[39] Caspar Pfeffinger and Jean Hermann were known primarily for their Jacobin zeal.[40] Hermann was soon replaced by Pierre Gorcy, an equally zealous military physician since 1791, who had risen to physician in chief of the armies of the Rhine and of the Sambre-et-Meuse.[41]

Among the six assistants appointed to the Strasbourg school were two who were to become great military surgeons under Napoleon. C. A. Lombard had been with the Army of the Rhine as a surgeon since 1791, and Bernard Bérot, a former student of Corvisart, had been a surgeon first class with the Army of the Côtes de Brest.[42] Lombard replaced Busch as an assistant professor on January 7, 1795. At the same time, Jean Roederer was named to assist Coze.[43] The oddest appointee was Antoine Barbier. A Jacobin who had renounced the priesthood and married in 1793, he had been in charge of the national depots and had served on the Committee of Public Education in 1794. His qualifications for assisting Flamant in surgery, gynecology, and pediatrics apparently rested upon a brief period as a military health officer.[44]

Each of the three medical schools took on its own particular characteristics. Paris was in the hands of the greatest civilian talents in clinical medicine, Montpellier was returned to most of its old faculty who were inclined toward theoretical medicine, and Strasbourg resumed its tradition of practical medicine. Yet all three reflected an important mingling of the old and new in medicine and surgery. The Committee of Public Safety insisted that the schools have the same curriculum and organization. Though the Committee required that the old Hippocratic course on fevers and old methods of healing be taught, there were some strikingly new courses.[45] Hygiene and prophylaxis were courses entirely new to the curriculum. Legal medicine consisted of five courses which embodied the knowledge gained from the wars since 1792: wounds in general, wounds of the head, wounds of the chest, wounds of the abdomen, and wounds of the extremities.[46] The old course that demonstrated the use of drugs and surgical instruments was split into two up-to-date courses. The school librarians were required to give an annual course on bibliography, indicating to students the best works on each aspect of medicine, the authors, and the latest editions.[47]

The shortage of qualified medical students continued to hamper the new schools, however. By February 24, the Committee of Public Safety opened the way for "citizens of the French colonies, whether natives or westerners" to be considered for admission.[48] The faculties were ordered to prepare an entrance examination which could be given to anyone appearing at the school and requesting admission. Each school director was instructed to notify the Committee of Public Education as to which districts had not yet sent students and which students had not yet arrived. The professors were authorized, as soon as this notification had been given to the Committee of Public Education, to begin examining replacements without regard to districts and to accept students up to the limit of the enrollment set by the Law of 14 Frimaire. When all vacancies were filled, any remaining applicants were to be placed on a waiting list.[49]

The military medical implications of this struggle to launch the new medical schools were evident and urgent. The Paris faculty initially acquired the building of the old Academy of Surgery (now the Ancienne Faculté Rue de l'Ecole de Médecine). With so many students to be accommodated, however, additional facilities were immediately required. Consequently, on January 10, 1795, the Committee of Public Safety gave the Commission of Arms and Powder just ten days to clear out of the old Cordeliers building so that the Paris school could have the space.[50]

When Plaichard and Barailon had difficulty getting faculty and space at Strasbourg, the Committee promptly intervened to assign professors from the armies, to allow multipurpose rooms for instruction, to require students to attend classes, to order professors not to loaf or distract the students, and to chide the local citizenry to "get busy and not obstruct things." It was concerned that "harmony [should] reign among the professors," so that "Strasbourg will constantly furnish health officers for our armies, which have the greatest need for them."[51] On March 10, the Committee of Public Safety set the month of Thermidor as the time for general examinations when the avancés could be graduated for immediate service with the armies. To spur the students to progress rapidly to this classification, it was decreed that anyone failing to pass the examination in Thermidor would be replaced and, if any of the failing students had been among the draftees of 1793, they would be returned to the army as "cowardly deserters."[52]

At about the same time (March 9), the Committee of Public Safety authorized the resumption of medical training at some private medical schools, such as the one at Caen. Financial assistance was given to get private institutions underway again, staffed by professors who could meet the test of having been classified as faculty in October of 1793.[53] These cases where civilian medical schools were allowed to reopen were exceptional, however, and each was subject to a policy decision by the Committee of Public Safety. By far the most promising private instruction was that in military medicine that began in Paris in late May of 1795 at Val-de-Grâce. The president of Val-de-Grâce was Coste, the medical inspector of military hospitals. Larrey was professor of anatomy and surgical operations. Another brilliant military surgeon, Nicolas Desgenettes, taught botany, chemistry, and medical materials.[54] On the authorization of the Convention in its law of August 7, 1793, military medical schools were soon established at Lille, Metz, and Toulon. Thus, once under way, the creation of facilities for medical training progressed rapidly during 1795 and 1796.

While pushing the staffing and equipping of the new schools of medicine and seeing to it that instruction commenced, the Committee of Public Safety was trying to cope with other problems of military medicine. Despite an acute lack of horses, the Committee ordered more carriages built for transporting the wounded and the sick.[55] Food was so short that many health officers killed their horses to feed their patients. Other health officers, the committee discovered, were selling their mounts and pocketing the proceeds.[56] In the Pyrenees, starving, shoeless troops cut up their haversacks to wrap their feet. On January 20, 1795, Amsterdam was finally taken in a blinding snowstorm by ten "shoeless, virtually nude" battalions of sick troops.[57] Epidemic fevers were rampant again as the winter's privations took their toll of resistance to disease. Drugs were so scarce that the Committee hastily dispatched the pharmacist Chalant to Belgium to make mass drug purchases for the armies.[58] Funds, equipment, and supplies were so wanting that some representatives on mission tried to conceal the fact that many hospitals were not even operating.[59]

The Committee of Public Safety had to lay down some ironclad rules to control the spread of epidemic diseases and to stop desertion from the hospitals. After January 8, 1795, sick soldiers could not go outside a hospital without a pass "issued for only the most indispensable and urgent reasons" signed by the police only after clearance by the chief health officer and the hospital director. The Committee further ordered that if there were a fan available to bring fresh air in to the patients, absolutely no patient could walk outside the hospital building.[60] An upsurge of venereal disease in the military hospitals produced another decree by the Committee, which again sought to regulate the presence of women in military establishments. The committee's decree flatly forbade any woman to live in a military hospital, but the exceptions the decree granted opened the way for subterfuge and evasion on a large scale and ruined its effectiveness. Like so many decrees before it, the January 28 decree made no real headway against the problem of venereal disease.[61]

Hoping to provide a definitive organization for military medicine, the Committee of Public Safety revived part of Carnot's plan of March 30, 1794. This short-lived piece of legislation had charged a Commission of Public Assistance with the full responsibility for administering, supplying, and financing all aspects of both civilian and military medicine.[62] The Committee also resurrected parts of the Laws of April 27, 1792, and of February 24, 1794 (Law of 3 Ventôse), which had continued, more or less, to govern military medicine.[63] A system foreshadowing a return to that of the Old Regime emerged in the Committee's decree of January 7, 1795. By its provisions, control of physicians, surgeons, and apothecaries in the military service passed from the hands of representatives of the Committee of Public Safety into the hands of paid civilian agents once again. Medical men kept their rank, pay, and hierarchical organization as provided for in the law of April 27, 1792, but they lost permanently any influence over administration, supply, and funds.[64]

Marking the assumption of national responsibility for supporting all hospitals, the January 7, 1795, decree of the Committee of Public Safety provided for all hospital costs to be paid from the national treasury. The Commission of Public Assistance was given full responsibility for the allocation of funds to hospitals, both civilian and military. Civilian hospitals would have their funds paid and their supplies drawn at the direction of the Commission of Public Assistance.[65]

Under the supervision of the commission, control of all military hospitals was given to a Central Agency of Military Hospitals. Composed of six members named by the Committee of Public Safety, the Central Agency consisted of Duroux and Mouron, who had been agents in charge of military hospitals of the armies of the Alps and the Sambre-et-Meuse, a former hospital administrator named Gouges, and three others.[66] The Central Agency was responsible for creating, maintaining, and administering all military hospitals, both fixed and mobile. The January 7 decree made the six members of the Central Agency "collectively responsible" and required that all records, supply orders, and drafts on the national treasury be signed by at least two of them.[67]

The Central Agency of Military Hospitals was to direct the military Hospital Service through its own paid agents. Potentially, the latter were little more than a revival of the old war commissioners.[68] A built-in safeguard against fraud, however, provided that military hospital funds, when authorized by the Central Agency and approved by the Commission of Public Assistance, were to be paid through the army paymasters.[69] Each agent nominated by the Central Agency had to be approved by the Commission or by the Committee of Public Safety. The Central Agency was held responsible for a prompt and proper accounting by all of its employees and was required to scrutinize all requests from them and review all receipts and disbursements on a trimester basis. The agents employed by the Central Agency were to be carefully supervised by several bureaus set up and controlled by the Central Agency, upon approval of the Commission of Public Assistance. For example, Gouges became director-general of the bureau of accounts. The law required that any agents found guilty of financial abuses were to be reported by Gouges directly to the Committee of Public Safety for punitive action.[70]

No purchases for military medicine could be made, however, except upon authorization by a separate Commission of Supply. The Law of January 7 gave the Commission of Supply full power to buy all provisions and equipment for the army medical service. For example, army mobile hospitals were to be supplied through each army's central supply depot and its subdepots but only upon proper authorization from the Commission of Supply. In charge of each central depot was an agent of the Commission of Supply, a quartermaster general who ranked as an equal of the Central Agency's agent for military hospitals. The subdepots were staffed by assistant quartermasters general who were ranked and paid as equals of hospital directors and physicians and surgeons first class.[71]

The Central Agency of Military Hospitals was required to ascertain the needs of the military medical service and to report these needs to the Commission of Public Assistance. The latter was responsible in turn for forwarding this information to the Commission of Supply. Purchases by the Central Agency and any of its agents were forbidden except when they were specifically authorized by the Commission of Supply or when the commission delegated to the Central Agency the power to buy some small items locally for local consumption. Even in such cases, however, the Central Agency was held strictly accountable for following the purchasing and accounting procedures of the Commission of Supply.[72]

The January 7, 1795, decree also established in each army an Agency of Hospitals, composed of an agent of the Central Agency, a director general, and a number of assistant directors.[73] In the jurisdiction of each army, every military hospital was given an administration composed of a director, an admissions commissioner, a commissioner of accounts, one or two clerks (depending upon the size of the hospital), a supply quartermaster, a paymaster, and a quartermaster in charge of the weapons, equipment, and personal effects of the patients. Every hospital with more than 500 patients enjoyed an additional employee, who was ranked and paid equally with the admissions commissioner. His function was to relieve the director of some supervisory duties and to assist with the office work. The army mobile hospitals and certain frontier hospitals were also assigned evacuation commissioners, who were responsible for accompanying convoys of patients from one hospital to another and who were authorized to "procure en route all of the assistance that the patients are due."[74] The law that still governed medical officers (Law of 3 Ventôse, an II) was cited as the standard that would govern the rank and pay of the hospital administrative personnel. Hospital directors, for example, were ranked and paid equally with military physicians and surgeons first class.[75]

Very shortly the obviously awkward position of the Central Agency of Military Hospitals was partially corrected. It quickly became apparent that the Commission of Public Assistance had too many responsibilities. Also the cumbersome machinery of the decree of January 7, which put the commission in an intermediary position between the Central Agency and the Commission of Supply, worked too slowly for wartime conditions. The system had various built-in checks against graft and corruption, but it failed to be responsive to urgent needs. Finally, the separation of military hospital administration from the rest of the military medical service produced endless confusion. The Commission of Health, composed of Fourcroy, Plaichard, and Barailon, was as deeply involved with military hospitals as was the new Central Agency.

To remedy these difficulties, a fifteen-member Council of Health was created by the Law of 12 Pluviose, an III (January 31, 1795). With Coste as chairman, the other physicians were Lorentz, Sabatier, DeBrest, and Beçu. The five surgeons named were Heurteloup, Villarle, Groffier, Saucerotte, and Buffin, and the pharmacists were Bayen, Parmentier, Hégo, Pelletier, and Brougniart. The Council assumed full responsibility for all military medicine. It reunited the administration of military hospitals with the administration of other aspects of military medicine. Under the Law of January 31, the Council could deal directly with the national treasury and with the Commission of Supply on all medical needs. The administrative hierarchy set up for military hospitals by the Law of January 7 was retained and its authority extended to govern medical personnel in the armies. The Council of Health thus acquired supervisory personnel through whom it could regulate military medical men according to the Law of April 27, 1792, and the military hospitals by the law of January 7, 1795. This was the organization of military medicine that the Convention bequeathed to the Directory.[76]

When the National Convention was dissolved on October 26, 1795, and the day of the Committees of Public Safety ended, the military medical organization was still unsettled. The Directory confined itself to a return to the prerevolutionary system of contracting for medical services. The Law of 31 Floréal, an IV (May 19, 1796) created *commissioner-ordonnateurs* who were given combined powers of administration, purchase, and supply, a system that encouraged in the military medical service a condition of renewed negligence and corruption.[77] This return to an old system "that allowed men to make a profit out of war" marked the end of experimentation that had sought to find a better system. Just as they had done before 1789, French military medical men once again bitterly condemned the contracting system, but to no avail. It endured throughout the Napoleonic era until it was ended by Louis XVIII.[78]

NOTES

1. Guillaume, *Convention* 5: xli. Fourcroy had been Marat's replacement in the Convention. Plaichard had been a moderate in both the Legislative Assembly and in the Convention, while Barailon had come to the Convention as a believer in "liberty without license" and sought to maintain a moderate position also. Both had voted against the death decree for Louis XVI.

2. Ibid., 5: 315; Aulard, *Recueil des actes* 15: 132; *Moniteur* 23: 85.

3. Cabanès, *Chirurgiens et blessés* p.338.

4. Guillaume, *Convention* 5: 334.

5. Ibid.

6. Ibid., 5: xlii, 375.

7. Ibid., 4: 980; 5: 282; Aulard, *Recueil des actess, 15: 132; Moniteur* 23: 618, 663–67.

8. Guillaume, *Convention* 5: 316, 323; Aulard, *Recueil des actes* 19: 149, 354–55; 21: 173, 263, 424; 22: 293, 649.

9. When Manoury elected to stay at the Hôtel-Dieu, the Committee of Public Safety replaced him on December 29 with Claude Pinson (1746? –1828), a former surgeon-major of the Swiss Guards (1777) and a military surgeon since 1792. Pinson dossier, carton 212, Val-de-Grâce. See also Aulard, *Recueil des actes* 19: 149.

10. Guillaume, *Convention* 5: 323—24; Aulard, *Recueil des actes* 21: 424; 22: 649.

11. On December 28, Montabret was replaced by Victor Broussonnet as professor of operative surgery and René Bertin was named as his assistant. See Guillaume, *Convention* 5: 373. Although given in Guillaume as Berthe, this is René Joseph Hyacinthe Bertin (1767—?) of Montpellier, a graduate of the medical school there, who served as a surgeon in the Army of the Côtes de Brest (1792—94), the Army of Italy (1796), was inspector-general of the health service (1798), and an army physician under Napoleon in Prussia and Poland (1807). Bertin dossier, carton 204 B/1, Val-de-Grâce. Victor Broussonnet (1771—1846), younger brother of the emigré physician Pierre Broussonnet, was one of the last to receive a medical degree at Montpellier in 1790. He served in the ambulance hospitals of the Army of the Eastern Pyrenees (1791—1795), Broussonnet dossier, carton 104B/II, ibid.

12. Guillaume, *Convention* 5: 355—56. Pfeffinger was replaced by Tinchant as curator on January 7, 1795; and, to replace Busch, C. A. Lombard was ordered from the Army of the Rhine to Strasbourg as assistant to Tourtelle, Lombard dossier, carton 109/1, Val-de-Grâce. Busch and Tinchant remain unknown and Caspar Pfeffinger, a Swiss Jacobin who fled to Strasbourg early in the Revolution, may have died shortly before January 7, 1795. See *Dict. encyclopédique sci. méd.* 2d ser., 23: 795.

13. Ackernecht, *Paris Hospital*, p.34.

14. *Nouvelle biographie* 23: 162. Jean Noël Hallé (1745—1822) of Paris, a famous civilian clinician.

15. Pelletan dossier, carton 212, Val-de-Grâce. Philippe Jean Pelletan (? —1829) was next in line to be surgeon-in-chief at the Hôtel-Dieu when Desault was given that position in 1785. He finally succeeded Desault in 1795. Pelletan might have been Napoleon's First Surgeon but Corvisart recommended Alexis Boyer. All of Pelletan's colleagues, except Desault who died in 1795, became barons of the Empire under Napoleon. See *Dict. encyclopédique sci. méd.*, 2d ser., 22: 393.

16. See above for biographical notes on Desault, Corvisart, and Chopart.

17. *Dict. encyclopédique sci. méd.*, 2d ser., 23: 786. Bernard Peyrilhe (1735—1804) of Perpignan.

18. Ibid., 2: 9. Pierre Lassus (1741—1807), member of the Council of Health, later a member of the Institute and Consulting Surgeon to Napoleon I.

19. See above for biographical note on Sabatier.

20. *Dict. encyclopédique sci. méd.*,1st ser., 30: 420—21. François Doublet (1751—95) of Chartres had been a physician at the Necker, at the Hôpital des Vénériens, and assistant inspector of civil hospitals in France during 1793—94.

21. See above for biographical note on Chaussier.

22. See above for biographical note on Fourcroy.

23. Leclerc dossier, carton 209/1, Val-de-Grâce. Claude Barthélemy Jean Leclerc served with the Army of the North, at the military hospital at St. Cyr, and then as assistant professor of clinical medicine at Paris. See Aulard, *Recueil des actes* 19: 355. See above for biographical note on Claude Pinson.

24. Armées du Nord, carton 26, Arch. hist. Service de Santé. Paul Augustin Olivier Mahon (1752–1801) of Chartres. See also *Dict. encyclopédique sci. méd.* 2d ser., 4: 2.

25. Antoine Dubois (1756–1837) of Gramat served with Napoleon in Egypt and wore the same costume all his life: a coat with huge sleeves, a short republican vest and tight pants of mid-calf length, Dubois dossier, carton 206/1, Val-de-Grâce. Alexis Boyer (1757–1833) of Uzerches (Corrèze), bourgeois, colorless but able, served with Napoleon in Prussia, Boyer dossier, carton 104 B/II, ibid.

26. See above for biographical note on Percy.

27. M. P. Lallement (d.1830) apparently was not distinguished, *Dict. encyclopédique sci. méd.* 2d ser., 1: 187. Louis Claude Richard (1754–1821) of Versailles had voyaged to Martinique, French Guiana, Guadaloupe, and Jamaica, returning to Paris in 1789. His lack of zeal for the Revolution made the years 1789–94 uncomfortable for him. Later, he was greatly esteemed and became a member of the Institute, ibid., 3d ser., 5: 16.

28. Ibid., 1st ser., 10: 424; 30: 605; 2d ser., 1:187; 4: 2.

29. Guillaume, *Convention* 5: 323–24. Spelled Beaumes by Guillaume, this is Jean Baptiste Timothée Baumes of Nîmes (1777–1828), *Nouvelle biographie* 4: 822. See also Jean Baumes, *Traité de la première dentition et des maladies souvent très-graves qui en dependent* (Paris, 1806), p.iii. René, who taught legal medicine, is known chiefly for his famous son, Gasparin Auguste René, who also taught legal medicine and succeeded his father at Montpellier, *Dict. encyclopédique sci. méd.*, 3d ser., 3: 389. Save for Antoine Gouan, the others are undistinguished. Broussonnet replaced Montabret on December 28, 1794. Guillaume, *Convention* 5: 373.

30. *Dict. encyclopédique sci. méd.* 1st ser., 15: 414–15.

31. Ibid., 4th ser., 9: 748–49. Antoine Gouan (1733–1821) of Montpellier, friend of Linnaeus, J. J. Rousseau, and a protégé of the Duc de Noailles.

32. Dumas dossier, carton 206/1, Val-de-Grâce. Charles Louis Dumas (1765–1813) of Lyon, member of the Royal Society of Medicine (1787). At one time, he courted Mlle. Julie Carron, the future mother of Jean Jacques Ampère. See André Marie Ampère, *Correspondance et souvenirs* (Paris, 1873), p.17, and *Dict. encyclopédique sci. méd.* 1st ser., 30: 652–53.

33. Lafabrie is unknown. J. M. J. Vigarous (n.d.) of Montpellier. His name is spelled incorrectly as Vigaroux by Aulard, *Recueil des actes* 19:

149, but is given correctly in Guillaume, *Convention* 5: 324 and in *Dict. encyclopédique sci. méd.* 5th ser., 3: 466.

34. *Nouvelle biographie* 5: 443; *Dict. encyclopédique sci. méd.* 1st ser., 3: 749.

35. Lorentz dossier, carton 209/1, Val-de-Grâce. Guillaume, *Convention* 5: 355—56, misspelled his name as Lorent aîne. It is given correctly in Aulard, *Recueil des actes* 19: 149 and in *Nouvelle biographie* 21: 643—44.

36. Lauth dossier, carton 209, Val-de-Grâce. Thomas Lauth (1758—1826) of Strasbourg, "one of the luminaries of the faculty at Strasbourg." *Dict. encyclopédique sci. méd.*, 2d ser., 2: 45.

37. Nicolas dossier, carton 210/2, Val-de-Grâce. Pierre Nicolas (1743—1816) of Nancy. Etienne Tourtelle (1756—1801) of Besançon received his medical degree at Montpellier in 1788. Among his many writings were his *Elemens d'hygiene*, 2 vols. (Strasbourg, 1797) and *Elemens de matière médicale* (Paris, 1802), Tourtelle dossier, carton 213/1, ibid.

38. Coze dossier, carton 205/1, Val-de-Grâce. Pierre Coze (1754—1822) of Ambleteuse.

39. Flamant dossier, carton 207/1, ibid. Pierre René Flamant 1762—1833) of Strasbourg. Guillaume, *Convention* 5: 355—56, misspelled his name as Flamand.

40. Hermann dossier, carton 207/3, Val-de-Grâce. Jean Hermann (1738—1800) of Barr in Alsace had been a professor at Strasbourg since 1769. He was given charge of gathering the collection of natural history into the national depot at Strasbourg during the Revolution. See *Dict. encyclopédique sci. méd.* 4th ser., 13: 609.

41. Gorcy dossier, carton 207/3, Val-de-Grâce. Pierre Christophe Gorcy (1758—1826), a student of Jadelot at Nancy and a protégé of J. P. Read at Metz before the Revolution. He later served in Italy, Holland, Syria, Germany, and Spain as a military physician.

42. Lombard dossier, carton 209/1, ibid. Claude Antoine Lombard of Dôle. Bernard Bérot's name is misspelled by Aulard, *Recueil des actes* 19: 149 as Béraud but is given correctly in Guillaume, *Convention* 5: 355—56. See Bérot dossier, carton 204 B/1, Val-de-Grâce.

43. Jean Roederer (1740—?) of Strasbourg had held the chair of anatomy there since 1767. Guillaume, *Convention* 5: 399; *Dict. encyclopédique Sci. méd.* 3rd ser., 5: 108.

44. Barbier dossier, carton 204 B/1, Val-de-Grâce, Antoine Alexandre Barbier (1765—1825), See also *Nouvelle biographie* 4: 443.

45. Guillaume, *Convention* 5: 502—3.

46. Laignel-Lavastine, *Histoire générale* 3: 469.

47. Guillaume, *Convention* 5: 502—3.

48. Ibid., 5:534.

49. Ibid.

50. Aulard, *Recueil des actes* 19: 394—95.

51. Guillaume, *Convention* 5: 493—94.

52. Ibid., 5: 591.

53. Ibid., 5: 570; McCloy, *Government Assistance*, p.441.

54. Larrey, *Memoirs* 1: 52, 60. Nicolas René Dufriche Desgenettes (1762—1837) of Alençon (Orne) received his degree at Montpellier in 1791, went to Italy to study, then returned to France in 1793 and served with the Army of Italy. At val-de-Grâce in 1795, he went with Napoleon to Egypt and later became a baron of the Empire. Desgenettes dossiers, cartons 202 bis and 202 ter, Val-de-Grâce.

55. Aulard, *Recueil des actes* 19: 579.

56. Ibid., 19: 361.

57. Cabanès, *Chirurgiens et blessés*, p.315.

58. Aulard, *Recueil des actes* 19: 395.

59. Ibid., 19: 591.

60. Ibid., 19: 359.

61. Ibid., 19: 728.

62. Ganges, *Représentants du peuple*, 1: 437—39.

63. See above, pp. 00, 000.

64. Aulard, *Recueil des actes* 19: 329—32.

65. Ibid., 19: 331.

66. Other than that given by Aulard, *Recueil des actes* 19: 383, no further information has been found on the Central Agency's personnel, possibly because it lasted only three weeks and may never have been fully formed.

67. Ibid., 19: 329—30.

68. Bottet, "Le passé," *Caducée* 5: 151.

69. Aulard, *Recueil des actes* 19: 331.

70. Ibid., 19: 332.

71. Ibid., 19: 331.

72. Ibid., 19: 329—30.

73. Ibid. Salaries for agents of the Central Agency of Military Hospitals who were with the armies were set at 1,000 livres per month. The director-generals received 666 livres and their assistants, whose number was determined by the location of the army and the number of its divisions, were paid 500 livres per month.

74. Ibid., 19: 330.

75. Ibid. Directors were salaried at 400 livres per month; admissions commissioners at 300 livres; clerks, supply quartermasters and commissioners of accounts at 200 livres; paymasters at 166 livres; and quartermasters of arms and evacuation commissioners at 150 livres.

76. Rapports aux inspecteurs-généraux, carton 21, Arch. hist. Service de Santé.

77. *Dict. encyclopédique sci. méd.* 2d ser., 8: 100.

78. Bottet, "Le passé," *Caducée* 5: 152.

Chapter Eleven

THE MEDICAL REVOLUTION

Two important eighteenth-century signs of change that pointed toward a new medicine in the nineteenth were the growth of clinical medicine and the hospital reform movement. The former had its roots in the amphitheaters of military medicine where practical experience had always counted for more than the speculative theories of medicine. In civilian practice, the influence of Desault, Desbois de Rochefort, and Pichault de la Martinière shaped a clinical medicine that stressed the value of accurate observation and the anatomical basis of medicine. The hospital reform movement of the 1780s promised a gradual improvement of unbelievably bad conditions, provided local enlightenment and funds could be found for the task. Neither of these new developments offered hope for a revolutionary change in French medicine, however. Hospital reform was costly, and many were convinced that hospitals should be abolished rather than reformed. The clinical medicine that was taught offered no greater hope for radical change—it was too individualized and too limited in scope to gain broad, practical application as long as the old medicine was dominant.

The two great catalysts that precipitated a real revolution in French medicine were political revolution and war. The first years of the Revolution were catastrophic for the old organization of French medicine. For a variety of reasons that were compelling to the revolutionaries, medical institutions came under violent attack. The universities and medical schools were abolished by forces that were essentially anti-intellectual and egalitarian. An ideological climate that gave preeminence to equality and virtue pulled down the learned societies and academies, which could have no place in the new social structure because by nature they recognized the superiority of some men, and they pursued ends that were not necessarily moral. Therefore many majestic structures of the Old Regime were toppled, not the least of which were the Royal Society of

Medicine and the Royal Academy of Surgery.

The Revolution was equally disastrous for the hospitals. Disorders helped to dry up private philanthropy, taxes went unpaid, and hospital earnings from endowment fell off. In their haste to abolish feudal dues taxes, fees, and monopolies, the revolutionary assemblies destroyed the traditional financial bases for hospitals in France. The attack directed at ecclesiastical orders and lay groups for religious reasons fostered a widespread disruption of nursing services and hospital administration. Hospital conditions which had horrified observers in the 1780s grew worse during the early years of the Revolution. Although emergency loans and grants of money were authorized by the assemblies, these funds were never adequate. When purges of experienced hospital personnel resulted in their replacement by war widows and orphans, the hospital service declined in mid-1793 to a point lower than any that the Old Regime had known. Victims of epidemic illnesses and the wounded produced by wartime conditions inundated the demoralized health care facilities and completed the disaster that befell the old hospital system.

When the revolutionaries undertook to create a new public health policy, they laid a significant foundation stone for the structure of a more modern medicine. Linking the ideals of liberty and happiness with equality and health, the committees of Public Welfare wove the principle of national responsibility for public health into the fabric of the new society. Rather than serving the needs of the rich and privileged, thereafter medicine would have to serve the nation. Implicit in the new policy was the expectation of centralized control, new national institutions and organizations, uniform rules and regulations, and the financial support of the State to insure better health care for the masses.

In both the destruction of the old system and the formulation of new policies of health and education, liberal and radical physicians and surgeons played an important role. Supporting the Revolution in great numbers, on the local level they preached a concern for hygiene, helped to organize public health facilities, and tried to serve the needs of the people. Some of these republican doctors served in the departmental and national assemblies, influencing the decisions of committees on national policies. When war came, they rushed into the military medical corps and gave dedicated service to the Republic's citizen-soldiers. The core of revolutionary physicians and surgeons that was loyal to the Revolution provided the energy and zeal for democratizing French medicine and expanding its responsibility to the whole nation. During the five-year cessation of formal medical education, they engaged in the protracted debate over education, its content, organization, and goals. When the exigencies of war finally required the resumption of formal medical education, they actively influenced the new curriculum, structure, and aims of the medical schools. The political activity of the liberal doctors proved to be a significant force in the reshaping of medicine and its institutions.

When the Revolution broke out, French military medicine had already been paralyzed by the economies of 1788. Initially the revolutionary assemblies made little effort to provide an effective medical service for the armies, even though an impending war made this both reasonable and imperative. After hostilities opened, the attempt to recruit only experienced medical men collapsed because the Revolution made no distinction among "health officers" so long as they all held licenses, easily purchased. In the same way that undisciplined and defective volunteers poured into the army battalions of 1792, incompetent and untrained practitioners flooded the medical service. The initiative for some sort of medical training was simply left to dedicated men, such as Coste, Larrey, Lorentz, and Percy, whose impromptu courses during campaigns involved herculean efforts to hold up some standard of medical care for the armies.

The failure of the assemblies to create a regular organization for the medical service appeared at first to be a blessing. It facilitated the reunion of medicine and surgery by lumping all medical men into the democratic category of "health officer." This permitted both surgeons and pharmacists to make good their claims to equality with physicians. Furthermore, once war was underway the Legislative Assembly's weak effort at organization appeared to herald a real golden age, because the medical service was freed from accountability and surveillance by the old war commissioners. Primarily as an act of expediency, military commanders were simply ordered to requisition and confiscate supplies for the medical men, and the latter were held responsible for fashioning somehow an effective medical system based upon this haphazard arrangement.

The attempt by medical men and army commanders to create a military medical system was heroic, but ultimately futile. With no funds, little organization, and few supplies and equipment, this impromptu arrangement simply could not meet the demands placed upon it. Medical men were confronted with a new type of warfare that was stupefying to all but the most hardened and experienced physicians and surgeons. Armies became great masses of men. Epidemic illnesses raced through their ranks with devastating effects. The hordes of armed French patriots sustained shocking battle casualties because of their inexperience and zeal. Charges in the face of artillery firing at point-blank range, such as the one at Aywaille, left frightful and needless carnage for the medical service to try to handle. The price of the Revolution's demand that generals win battles at all costs was appalling in terms of the human losses involved. The organized system of military medicine that had belonged to the Old Regime could not have handled such terrifying numbers of sick and wounded; much less could the improvised medical service of 1792.

The chaotic state into which military medicine had fallen by mid-1793 required ruthless measures to correct. The force and intimidation that had to be applied to mobilize France for total war and survival had to be levied against military medicine as well. If the urgent needs of the sick and wounded were to be met, the lack of a regular medical organization, the exhaustion of medical supplies and equipment, and the shortage of health officers had to be remedied by emergency political action from Paris. Negligence and incompetence were equated with treason, and carelessness was severely punished on the spot. The physicians and surgeons who survived the terrible years of 1793 and 1794 had to accommodate the centralized authority and iron discipline of the Committee of Public Safety. Supported by popular concern for the nation's sick and wounded defenders, benefiting from the zeal and dedication of Jacobin medical men, and displaying no reluctance to take complete control of military medicine, the Committee of Public Safety strongly influenced the future of French medicine by the pressures it brought to bear upon the wartime practice of medicine and surgery.

The war produced some profound changes in medicine. On the battlefield, the untested teachings of civilian medicine proved to be faulty and ineffective. Many of the complicated medicines and techniques of speculative medicine were either simplified or abandoned. The inability of the physician trained in "library" medicine to cope with the wounds and epidemic diseases of wartime severely damaged his prestige. His medical role changed from that of a superior to that of a colleague of the surgeon, from whom he had much to learn about practical medicine. This cooperation between physician and surgeon, each bearing the democratic title of "health officer," provided a climate that hastened the reunion of medicine and surgery.

With great numbers of untrained or mediocre medical practitioners in military service; there was unparalleled opportunity and necessity for them to become anatomists. The physician soon found himself considered useless unless he changed his ways; he did not possess the surgeon's indispensable skill, and he discovered that the surgeon was quite willing to prescribe and care for his patients. Many, in fact, emphatically expressed their preference for the surgeon. The physician, overwhelmed by epidemic illnesses, forced to use simple medicinals, threatened by political agents, and spurred by aggressive and inventive surgeons, had every incentive to adopt the surgeon's point of view.

The fact that many physicians dropped their speculative medical theories and embraced the localized pathology of the surgical approach to medicine is of profound significance. As autopsies became routine, the causes of illness came to be seen concretely in the tumors, abscesses, ulcers, inflammations, and hemorrhages located inside the body. Thus, a new concept of disease was evolving. The common approach to medicine shared by physicians and surgeons based upon anatomy and local pathology was an outcome of wartime pressures that changed the whole medical outlook for the future.

The wartime emergency forced health officers to practice in much the same way that army commanders were fighting: use what they had and expect no help. Usually without much equipment, military surgeons learned to do wonders with simple pocket scalpels, probes, tweezers, and, if necessary their fingers. They became masters of the bandage, primarily because it could be ingeniously adapted to many purposes and could often compensate for the lack of surgical supplies. Many harmful practices in French medicine were quickly controlled or eliminated by experience with battlefield conditions. The abuse of wound excision, for example, was exposed when hemorrhaging came to be better understood, and compression was abandoned as a means of dealing with massive hemorrhages because it was not suited to wartime conditions.

Ingenuity and improvisation became indispensable assets for French medical men during the critical war years. Skin grafts were still unknown, but experimenters such as Briot successfully reapplied skin fragments sliced off by sabres. In a moment of inspiration, it was Sabatier who showed his surgeons how a severed intestine could be sutured when drawn together over an ordinary rolled-up playing card. Larrey demonstrated catheterization as a new and remarkably effective way to treat bladder wounds. The technique of putting a patient in a drunken stupor before setting a bone was common, but it was inadequate for setting pelvic bones and broken hips. Military medicine soon learned from simple country practitioners that relaxation of the great muscles of the legs and abdomen could be secured by the narcotic effect of simply inserting a strong cigar into the rectum.

The shortage of medicines, supplies, and equipment during the war actually contributed to an improvement in the treatment of wounds and disease. Mercifully, after 1792 greasy ointments and perfumed solutions were no longer readily available. Because nothing else was available, plain water was frequently the only medication that could be applied to even the most serious wounds. Larrey originated wound irrigation, and experience proved the superiority of water's healing qualities. Lack of sutures and needles led to Larrey's discovery of healing by "union of third intention," the simple practice of holding wound edges together by proper bandaging.

Battlefield conditions required an approach to wounds that emphasized speed and practicality. The tourniquet and cautery iron gave way to the practice of seizing an open vein, pulling it up and tying it off. Battle situations often forced quick amputations. Larrey anticipated a modern technique by trying refrigeration to ease the terrible pain of amputations. In pre-anesthesia days, the demand for speed helped to improve and simplify amputations. More suitable points for amputation, better stumps to match the newly developed artificial limbs, and improved post-operative care for amputees emerged from the experience of thousands of wartime amputations. Larrey's rule that amputation should be done within 24 hours became the standard guide in French military medicine because it was practical and speedy. The fortunate corollary of this 24-hour rule was that remarkably fewer men were lost to gangrene and tetanus.

One of the valuable resources of the new medicine in France was the prolific outpouring of hospital reports, special studies by individual physicians and surgeons, and memoranda of all sorts detailing medical problems and solutions. Full of statistical information, autopsy results, and observations on a wide variety of wounds and diseases, the wartime literature of medicine created a rich resource of thousands upon thousands of painstakingly compiled case studies. From these raw materials, the textbooks of a new medicine would be drawn, and the discoveries and lessons of the war years would be transmitted to civilian medicine.

Although clinicians such as Corvisart, Desault, and Pinel were powerful influences upon the rise of hospital medicine, it was the war and the thinking of military medical men which forced widespread acceptance of the hospital as the key medical institution of the future. From 1792 and the time of Percy's and Larrey's concern for speedy evacuation of wounded men, the hospital had presented itself as the only logical way to serve the medical needs of the armies. Mass casualties and the incredible numbers of soldiers felled by epidemic diseases and other ailments could not have been handled by the small number of medical men except in a central place—a hospital equipped and staffed for that purpose. Backed by the popular demand that proper medical care be given to the soldiers of the Republic, medical men and political representatives competed in trying to establish hospitals everywhere.

The Revolution's acceptance of the hospital as the basic medical institution was highly significant. No longer just a place of care, the new hospitals were conceived as true medical centers concerned with treatment, cure, and teaching. They were readily integrated into the goal of free public health care, and because of national financing, the hospitals could be centrally controlled and subjected to standardized rules and improved procedures. Enlightened concerns for sanitation, hygiene, vaccination, ventilation, and private beds were now enforceable in a national system. The hospitals themselves offered the best framework for practicing the new medicine. Their autopsy rooms, statistical compilations, and teaching staffs were the supports of improved diagnosis and treatment. Hospital-centered medicine, on a nationwide basis, was truly one of the most important developments of the Revolution and the war.

When medical education was finally reinstituted by the convention in 1795, it was a purely pragmatic move dictated by critical national needs. The ideological deadlock on public education remained, but the pressing urgency for more medical men could not wait. The structure of the new "schools of health," the make-up of their staffs, and the lip-service paid to Hippocrates and Galen in the curriculum, illustrated the post-Thermidorean tendency to reestablish links with the past. That Paris no longer dominated the Revolution was evident in the fact that Fourcroy's proposed 500-student medical school in Paris was modified to establish three schools in places where traditions for medical education were strong, Paris, Montpellier, and Strasbourg. The old faculty at Montpellier was virtually restored. At the Paris school, great figures of clinical medicine of the prerevolutionary days were selected as professors. Strasbourg was dominated by illustrious men from military medicine.

Despite these confusing appearances, the new medical schools reflected an important mingling of the best of the old and the new in French medicine, just as did the uniform curriculum prescribed by the Committee of Public Safety. The professors of medical chemistry were now teaching Lavoisier's principles rather than Stahl's discredited "phlogiston" theory. Entirely new courses were added to the program of studies, including hygiene, prophylaxis, and legal medicine. Because of the nature of the new field of legal medicine, the medical school faculties used it as a back door through which knowledge gained from the war could be brought into the classroom. To counteract some of the aspects of the required course in Hippocratic medicine, legal medicine was stretched to cover a multitude of medical and surgical areas, including five courses on wounds and wound treatments. Such a combination of the old and the new became the foundation for medical education in France after 1795.

In September of 1795, the Commission of Health addressed the following circular letter to all chief health officers of the French armies:

"You have won victory and national recognition. The infamous Coalition has succumbed to republican valor but, as the final blows are struck against our enemies, it is time to prepare to redouble our efforts on behalf of republican soldiers. Schools should be opened in all of the armies and, with the abundance of instructors we now have, the instruction of beginners undertaken. In the large hospitals, the physicians can teach medical chemistry. Demonstrations in anatomy and physiology can be given to all young surgeons. All republican hospital personnel ought to be in school, along with the health officers as their instructors in these medical courses; all should perfect their abilities or acquire new ones."[1]

A more revealing yet succinct statement would be difficult to find. The military medical service and its accomplishments during the critical years of 1792–1795 are recognized in the tone of confidence and praise. The strong sense of national obligation to the citizen-soldiers of the Republic is manifest. A strong and clear dedication to renewed medical education is evident, especially in the new medicine that was practical and hospital centered. The hospital, including its teaching function, is the natural medical center. Implicit in the statement is the goal of a public concern—that the great numbers of health officers and hospital personnel could upgrade their skills and train others in order to serve the larger needs of French society now that the war was coming to a close.

With the exception of a broad acceptance of the idea of contagion, the main outlines of the new hospital medicine of the nineteenth century were visible by 1796. It remained for the medical men who had survived the war and the students who would come out of the new medical schools to develop and perfect it. New challenges awaited them in Italy, Egypt, Syria, Santo Domingo, Spain, Germany, and Russia, and other medical discoveries and innovations were imminent. The Revolution allowed many brilliant but deprived boys the opportunity to enter the medical profession and to rise to eminence in it. They followed Napoleon loyally in far-flung campaigns and many of them were loaded with honors: Boyer, Desgenettes, Dubois, Larrey, and Péborde as barons of the Empire or Gorcy and Lombard in the Legion of Honor. Achieving a similar glory in civilian medicine were Broussais, the great hygienists Fodéré and Reveillé-Parise; Laënnec for the invention of the stethoscope, Bretonneau for the discovery of diphtheria, and Bichat for creating the science of histology.

Most significant was the effect of the wars and the new medicine upon the attitudes of the French people. The old attitudes of contempt, anger, and frustration toward medical men had changed. The knowledgeable, respected, and kindly physicians in the works of Balzac and Flaubert reflect the gratitude and admiration of their countrymen for the men of the medical profession. Perhaps there is no clearer indicator of how broad and deep were the changes in French medicine after 1789. In a way, it summarizes the fundamental achievements of the medical profession during the years that followed. This was no narrow technical revolution in medicine that had occurred; the change spread its influence across the spectrum of French life and letters. For all the loss, anguish, and destruction of the Revolution and the war, a new medicine had been born amidst the rubble of 1789—96, to which many Frenchmen literally owed their lives or their health and happiness.

NOTES

1. Conseil de Santé documents, carton 20, Arch. hist. service de Santé.

BIBLIOGRAPHY

References and Guides

Atkinson, James. *Medical Bibliography*. London: Churchill, 1834.

Augè, Paul. *Larousse du XXe siécle*. Paris: Librairie Larousse, 1931.

Bonnerot, Jean. *La Bibliothèque centrale et les archives du Service de Santé*. Paris: Librairie Ancienne Honoré Champion, 1918.

―――. *La Collection à l'autographes du Service de Santé du Musée Val-de-Grâce*. Paris: n.p., c.1918.

Deutsches Wörterbuch von Jacob Grimm und Wilhelm Grimm. 16 vols. Leipzig: Verlag von S. Hirzel, 1854–1960.

Dictionnaire de médecine, ou répertoire générale des sciences médicales considerées sous le rapport théorique et pratique par MM. Adelon et al. 2d ed. 30 vols. Paris: Béchet jeune, 1832–45.

Fondation Nationale des Sciences Politiques. *Elemens de bibliographie sur l'histoire des idées et des faits politiques, économiques, et sociaux depuis le milieu du XVIIIe siècle.* 2d ed., Paris: Domat-Montchréstien, 1948.

Gilbert, Judson Bennett. *Disease and Destiny: A Bibliography of Medical References to the Famous*. London: Dawsons, 1963.

Hawkins, Robert R., ed. *Scientific, Medical and Technical Books Published in the United States of America, 1930–1944: A Selected List of Titles in Print With Annotations*. Washington, D.C.: The National Research Council, 1950.

―――. *Supplement to Books Published, 1945–1948*. Washington, D.C.:

The National Research Council, 1950.

———. *Second Supplement of Books Published, 1949–1952*. Washington, D.C.: The National Research Council, 1953.

Hyamson, Albert M. *A Dictionary of Universal Biography of All Ages and of All Peoples*. New York: E. P. Dutton, 1951.

Hyslop, Beatrice F. "Les cahiers de doléances de 1789." *Annales historique de la Révolution française* 27: 115–23.

———. "French Historical Periodicals." *American Historical Review* 52 (1947): 369–71.

———. *Guide to the General Cahiers of 1789*. New York: Columbia University Press, 1936.

———. "Historical Publications Since 1939 on the French Revolution." *Journal of Modern History* 20 (1948): 232–50.

———. "Recent Works on the French Revolution." *American Historical Review* 47 (1942): 488–517.

Jones, Harold W.; Hoerr, Normand L.; and Osol, Arthur. *Blakiston's New Gould Medical Dictionary*. Philadelphia: The Blakiston Co., 1949.

Montfalcon, Jean Baptiste. *Précis de bibliographie médicale, contenant l'indication et la classification des ouvrages les meilleurs, les plus utiles, la description des livres de luxe et des éditions rares, et des tables pour servir à l'histoire de la médecine*. Paris: Baillière, 1827.

Morton, Leslie T. *Garrison and Morton's Medical Bibliography*. 2d ed. London: Argosy, 1961.

Palmer, Robert Roswell. "Bibliographical Article: Fifty Years of the Committee of Public Safety." *Journal of Modern History* 13 (1941): 375–97.

Pauly, A. *Bibliographie des sciences médicales*. London: Academic and Bibliographical Publications, 1954.

Reynolds Historical Library. "The Medical Library of Dr. Lawrence Reynolds." 2 vols. Unpublished manuscript. Birmingham, Ala.: University of Alabama Medical Center, 1960.

United States Army. *Index-Catalogue of the Library of the Surgeon-General's Office*. 1st ser. (1880–95), 16 vols.; 2d ser. (1896–1916), 21 vols.; 3d ser. (1918–32), 10 vols.; 4th ser. (1936–55), 11 vols.; 5th ser. (1959–61), 3 vols. Washington, D. C.: Government Printing Office, 1880–1961.

U. S. Department of Health, Education and Welfare, National Library of Medicine. *Bibliography of Medical Translations* Supplements 1–8. Bethesda, Md.: 1965.

———. *Bibliography of the History of Medicine*. 3 vols. Bethesda, Md.: 1965–67.

Manuscript Collections

Paris Archives historique du Service de Santé militaire.
———. Archives nationales, Acquisitions française.
———. Bibliothèque nationale. Fonds française.
———. Musée Val-de-Grâce.
Vincennes. Archives historique de l'armée.

Sources

Ampère, André Marie. *Correspondance et souvenirs (de 1793 à 1805)*. 5th ed. Paris: J. Hetzel, 1873.

Aulard, Alphonse, ed. *Recueil des actes du Comité de salut public*. 26 vols. Paris: Imprimerie nationale, 1889–1923.

Baumes, Jean Baptiste Timothée. *Traité de la première dentition et des maladies souvent très-graves qui en dépendent*. Paris: Méquignon l'aîme, 1806.

Bichat, Xavier. *Pathological Anatomy: The Last Course of Xavier Bichat, from an autographic manuscript of P. A. Béclard; with an account of the Life and Labours of Bichat by F. G. Boisseau*. Translated by Joseph Togno. Philadelphia: John Grigg, 1827.

———. *Recherches physiologiques sur la vie et la mort*. 2d ed. Paris: Librairie Brosson et Gabon et Cie., an X [1802] .

———. *Traité des membranes en générale et des diverses membranes en particulier*. Paris: Richard, Caille et Ravier, an VIII [1800].

Bloch, Camille, and Tuetey, Alexandre, eds. *Procès-verbaux et rapports du Comité de Mendicité de la Constituante, 1790–1797 (Collections de documents inédits sur l'histoire économique de la Révolution française publié par le Ministère de l'Instruction Publique)*. Paris: Imprimerie nationale, 1911.

Bordeu, Théophile de. *Recherches sur quelques points d'histoire de la médecine*. Liège: n.p., 1764.

Briot, Pierre François. *Histoire de l'état et des progrès de la chirurgie militaire en France pendant les guerres de la Révolution*. Besançon: Gautier, 1817.

Brocklesby, Richard. *Oeconomical and Medical Observations Tending to the Improvement of the Military Hospitals, and to the Cure of Camp Diseases, Incident to Soldiers*. London: T. Becket and P. A. DeHondt, 1764.

Cabanis, Peter John George. *On the Degree of Certitude in Medicine.* Translated by R. La Roche. Philadelphia: R. Desilver, 1828.

Chémant, Nicolas Dubois de. *Dissertation sur les avantages des nouvelles dents et rateliers artificiels, incorruptibles et sans odeur, inventés.* Paris: Librairie Gattey, 1789.

Clémanceau, Joseph. "Notes sur les Etats-Généraux et l'Assemblée constituante." *Revue historique de la Révolution française* 12 (1917): 129.

Clendening, Logan, ed. *Source Book of Medical History.* New York: P. B. Hoeber, 1942.

Cochin, Augustin, and Charpentier, Charles, eds. *Les actes du gouvernement Révolutionnaire (23 août 1793–27 juillet 1794). Recueil de documents publiés pour la Société d'histoire contemporaine.* 3 vols. Paris: Librairie Alphonse Picard et Fils, 1920–35.

Dictionnaire encyclopédique des sciences médicales, publié sous la direction de MM. les docteurs Raige-Delorme et A. Deschambre, par MM. les docteurs Axenfeld, Baillarger et al. 1st ser. (A–E), 36 vols.; 2d ser. (L–P), 27 vols.; 3rd ser. (Q–T), 18 vols.; 4th ser. (F–K), 16 vols.; 5th ser. (U–Z), 3 vols. Paris: P. Asselin, Sr. de Labé, V. Masson et Fils, 1864–89.

Diderot, Denis. *Encyclopédie des sciences: Chirurgie.* Paris: n.p., 1780.

Dumas, Charles Louis. *Systeme méthodique de nomenclature et de classification des muscles du corps humaine.* Paris: n.p., 1797.

France. *Edit du Roy, portant création d'Offices de Conseillers de Sa Majesté, Médecins et Chirurgiens Inspecteurs Généraux, et Majors à la suite des armées, dans tous les Hôpitaux, Villes Frontières, et anciens Régiments. Donné à Versailles, au mois de janvier 1708.* Paris: Imprimerie royale, 1708.

———. *Edit du Roy, portant suppression des charges de Médecins et de Chirurgiens, crées par Edit du mois de janvier 1708. Donné à Paris, au mois de juin 1716.* Paris: Imprimerie royale, 1716.

———. *Formules de médicaments rédigées dans la Conseil de Santé des hôpitaux militaires par ordre du Conseil de Guerre.* Paris: Imprimerie royale, 1788.

———. *Formules de pharmacie pour les hôpitaux militaires du Roy.* Paris: Imprimerie royale, 1747.

———. *Loi relatif aux officiers privés de leur état sans cause légitime ou arbitrairement suspendus de leur fonctions depuis 12 septembre 1791.* Paris: Imprimerie Nationale exécutive du Louvre, 1793.

———. *Programme des cours révolutionnaires sur l'art militaire, l'administration militaire, la santé des troupes et les moyens de conserver–fait aux élèves de l'Ecole de Mars depuis le 5 fructidor jusqu'au 13 vendémaire an III de la République.* Paris: Imprimé par ordre de Comité de Salut Public, 1793.

———. *Règlement fait par ordre du roi, pour établir dans les Hôpitaux militaires de Strasbourg, Metz, et Lille, des ampithéâtres destinés à former en médecine, chirurgie et pharmacie, des Officiers de santé pour le service des Hôpitaux militaires du royaume et des armées. Du 22 septembre 1775.* Paris: Imprimerie royale, 1775.

———. Convention Nationale, *Projet d'éducation du peuple française, presenté à la Convention nationale par Joseph Lakanal.* Paris: Imprimerie nationale, 1793.

Franklin, Benjamin. *Report of Benjamin Franklin and Other Commissioners Charged by the King of France With the Explanation of Animal Magnetism.* London: J. Johnson, 1785.

Ganges, Bonnal de. *Les représentants du peuple en mission près les armées, 1791–1797.* 4 vols. Paris: A. Savaète, 1898.

Guillaume, M. J., ed. *Procès-verbaux du Comité d'instruction publique de l'Assemblée Législative.* Paris: Imprimerie nationale, 1889.

———. *Procès-verbaux du Comité d'instruction publique de la Convention nationale.* 6 vols. Paris: Imprimerie nationale, 1891–1904.

Howard, John. *An Account of the Principal Lazarettos in Europe; With Various Papers Relative to the Plague: Together With Further Observations on Some Foreign Prisons and Hospitals; and Additional Remarks on the Present State of Those in Great Britain and Ireland.* Warrington, England: W. Eyres, 1789.

Lafont-Gouzi, G. G. *Matériaux pour servir à l'histoire de la médecine militaire en France.* Paris: Librairie Gabon, 1809.

Larrey, Dominique Jean. *Memoirs of Military Surgery, and Campaigns of the French Armies on the Rhine, in Corsica, Catalonia, Egypt, and Syria; at Boulogne, Ulm, and Austerlitz; in Saxony, Prussia, Poland, Spain and Austria.* Translated by Richard Willmott Hall. 4 vols. Baltimore: Joseph Cushing, 1814.

———. *Recueil de mémoires de chirurgie.* Paris: Compère jeune, 1821.

———. *Relation historique et chirurgicale de l'expédition de l'armée d'orient, en Egypte et en Syrie.* Paris: Démonville et Souers, an XI [1803].

———. *Surgical Essays.* Translated by John Rovere. Baltimore: N. G. Maxwell, 1823.

Le Dran, Henri François. *Traité ou réflexions tirées de la pratique sur les playes d'armes à feu.* Paris: C. Osmont, 1737.

Madival, M. J., and Laurent, M. E., eds. *Archives parlementaires de 1787 à*

1860. Recueil complet des débats législatifs et politiques des chambres françaises (1787–1793), lere sèrie, 1787–1799. 82 vols. Paris: Paul Dupont, 1862–1919.

Marat, Jean Paul. *Découvertes de M. Marat sur la lumière.* Paris: Jombert, 1780.

——— . *Recherches physiques sur le feu.* Paris: Jombert, 1780.

——— . *Recherches physiques sur l'électricité; par M. Marat, Docteur en Médecine et Médecin des Gardes du Corps de Monseigneur le Comte d'Artois.* Paris: Clousier, 1782.

Morand, Sauveur François. *Catalogue des pièces d'anatomie, instrumens, machines &c. qui composent l'arsenal de chirurgie formé à Paris pour la Chancellerie de Médecine de Petersbourg.* Paris: Imprimerie royale, 1759.

Parè, Ambroise. *La manière de traicter les playes faictes tant par hacquebutes, que par flèches; et les accidentz d'icelles, comme fractures et caries des os, gangrène et mortification; avec les pourtraictz des instrumentz nécessaires pour leur curation. Et la méthode de curer les combustions principalement faictes par la pouldre à canon.* Paris: n.p., 1552. See also *The Apologie and Treatise of Ambroise Paré, Containing the Voyages Made Into Divers Places, With Many of His Writings Upon Surgery. Edited and with an Introduction by Geoffrey Keynes.* London: Falcon Educational Books, 1951.

Percy, Pierre François. *Journal des campaigns du baron Percy, chirurgien-en-chief de la grande armée (1754–1825), publié d'aprè les manuscrits inédits avec une introcution par M. E. Longin, etc.* Paris: Plon, 1904.

——— . *Manuel du chirurgien d'armée, ou instruction de chirurgie militaire sur le traitement des plaies, et spécialement de celles d'armes à feu; avec la méthode d'extraire de ces plaies les corps étrangers, et la description d'un nouvel instrument propre à cet usage. Ouvrage qui a remporté le prix au concours de l'Académie royale de chirurgie de Paris.* Paris: Méquignon, 1792.

Petit, Jean Louis. *A Treatise of the Diseases of the Bones; Containing an Exact and Compleat Account of the Nature, Signs, Causes, and Cures Thereof, in Representing All Their Various Kinds, as* [sic] *Also the Figures Representing the Several Dressings, Machines, and Instruments Here Described.* London: T. Woodward, 1726.

Pringle, John. *Observations on the Diseases of the Army.* London: A. Millar and D. Wilson, 1752.

Ravaton, Hugues. *Chirurgie d'armée.* Paris: P. F. Didot le jeune, 1768.

Réimpression de l'ancien Moniteur [universel] *seule histoire authentique et inaltérée de la Révolution française depuis la réunion des Etats-*

Généraux jusqu'au Consulat (mai 1789–novembre 1799), avec des notes explicatives. 32 vols. Paris: Plon Frères, 1847–50.

Société Royale de Médecine. *Projet d'instruction sur une maladie convulsive, fréquente dans les colonies de l'Amerique connue sous le nom de Tetanos.* Paris: Imprimerie royale, 1786.

Tennetar, Michel. *Traitement de la Dyssenterie qui régne dans le département de la Moselle (en Septembre 1793).* Metz: C. L'Amort, 1793.

Tenon, René. *Mémoires sur les hôpitaux de Paris.* Paris: n.p., 1788.

Thompson, J. M., ed. *French Revolution Documents, 1789–1794.* London: Blackwell, 1933.

Van Swieten, Gerard L. B. *The Diseases Incident to Armies, With the Method of Cure.* American edition. Philadelphia: R. Bell, 1776.

Vellay, Charles. "Autographes et documents." *Revue historique de la Révolution française* 11 (1917): 173; 12: 175.

Vidal, Pierre. "Cassanyes et ses mémoires inédits." *La Révolution française* 14: 968–1008.

———. "Documents inédits: mission de Cassanyes aux armées d'Italie et des Alpes réunies" *La Révolution française.* 11: 440–64, 540–66.

Young, Arthur. *Travels in France During the Years 1787, 1788, 1789.* Edited by M. Betham-Edwards. London: G. Bell and Sons, 1913.

Secondary Works

Ackernecht, Erwin H. *Medicine at the Paris Hospital, 1794–1848.* Baltimore: Johns Hopkins University Press, 1967.

Aulard, Alphonse. *Histoire politique de la Révolution française.* Paris: Librairie Armand Colin, 1926.

Baas, Johann Herman. *Outlines of the History of Medicine and the Medical Profession.* Translated by H. E. Handerson. New York: W. R. Jenkins, 1889.

Bon, Henri. *Laënnec, 1781–1826.* Dijon: Lumière, 1925.

Brinton, Crane. *A Decade of Revolution, 1789–1799.* Rise of Modern Europe Series. New York: Harper and Brothers, 1934.

———. *The Jacobins: An Essay in the New History.* New York: Russell and Russell, 1961.

Cabanès, Augustin. *Chirurgiens et blessés à travers l'histoire.* Paris: Albin Michel, 1918.

———. *Le costume du médecin en France de Molière à nos jours.* Paris: P.

Longuet, n.d.

———. *Les évadés de la médecine.* Paris: A. Michel, 1931.

———. *La médecine en caricature.* Paris: P. Longuet, n.d.

———. *Médecins amateurs.* Paris: A. Michel, 1932.

Clagett, Marshall, ed. *Critical Problems in the History of Science.* Proceedings of the Institute for the History of Science. Madison: University of Wisconsin Press, 1959.

Coleman, William. *Georges Cuvier, Zoologist: A Study in the History of Evolution Theory.* Cambridge: Harvard University Press, 1964.

Corlieu, Auguste. *Le centenaire de la Faculté de Médecine de Paris (1794–1894).* Paris: n.p., 1896.

Cox, Frederick H.; Weber, Bernerd C.; Brace, Richard M.; and Ramsey, John F., eds. *Studies in Modern European History in Honor of Franklin Charles Palm.* New York: Bookman Associates, 1956.

Cruchet, René. *Médecine et littérature.* Romance Language Series No. 2. University, La.: Louisiana State University Press, 1939.

Darnton, Robert. *Mesmerism and the End of the Enlightenment in France.* Cambridge: Harvard University Press, 1968.

Delaunay, Paul. *D'une révolution à l'autre, 1789–1848.* Paris: Jules Rousset, 1949.

Delorme, Edmond. *War Surgery.* Translated by Henri de Meric. London: H. K. Lewis, 1915.

D'Echevannes, Carlos. *La vie d'Ambroise Paré, père de la chirurgie, 1510–1590.* Vies des hommes illustrés, No. 52. Paris: Librairie Gallimard, 1930.

Fayet, Joseph. *La Révolution française et la science, 1789–1795.* Paris: Librairie Marcel Rivière, 1960.

Garrison, Fielding H. *Notes on the History of Military Medicine.* Washington: Association of Military Surgeons, 1922.

Gershoy, Leo. *From Despotism to Revolution, 1763–1789.* Rise of Modern Europe Series. New York: Harper and Row, 1963.

Greer, Donald. *The Incidence of the Emigration During the French Revolution.* Cambridge: Harvard University Press, 1951.

———. *The Incidence of the Terror During the French Revolution: A Statistical Interpretation.* Cambridge: Harvard University Press, 1935.

Grimaux, Edouard. *Lavoisier, 1743–1794, d'après sa correspondance, ses manuscrits, ses papiers de famille et d'autre documents inédits.* Paris: Ancienne Librairie Gormer Baillière et Cie., 1896.

Hampson, Norman. *A Social History of the French Revolution.* London: Routledge and Kegan Paul, 1963.

Hoefer, J. C. F., ed. *Nouvelle biographie générale depuis les temps plus reculés jusqu'à nos jours, avec les renseignements bibliographiques et l'indication des sources à consulter.* 46 vols. Paris: Didot, 1853–66.

King, Lester. *The Medical World of the Eighteenth Century.* Chicago: University of Chicago Press, 1958.

Kobler, John. *The Reluctant Surgeon: The Life of John Hunter.* London: Heinemann, 1960.

Laignel-Lavastine, Maxime. *Histoire générale de la médecine, de la pharmacie, de l'art dentaire, et de la vétérinaire.* 3 vols. Paris: A. Michel, 1936–49.

Laurent, Charles. *Histoire de la vie et des ouvrages de P. F. Percy, composée sur les manuscrits originaux.* Versailles: Imprimerie Daumont, 1827.

Lefebvre, Georges. *The French Revolution from its Origins to 1793.* Translated by Elizabeth Moss Evanson. London: Routledge and Kegan Paul, 1962.

–––. *The French Revolution from 1793–1799.* Translated by John Hall Stewart and James Friguglietti. New York: Columbia University Press, 1964.

Lemaire, L. *Historique de l'hôpital de Dunkerque.* Paris: Charles Lavauzelle, 1936.

Loomis, Stanley. *Paris in the Terror, June 1793–July 1794.* Philadelphia: J. B. Lippincott, 1964.

Mathiez, Albert. *The French Revolution.* Translated by Catherine Alison Phillips. New York: Knopf, 1929.

Mathison, Richard R. *The Eternal Search: The Story of Man and His Drugs.* New York: G. P. Putnam's Sons, 1958.

McCloy, Shelby Thomas. *French Inventions of the Eighteenth Century.* Lexington: University of Kentucky Press, 1952.

–––. *Government Assistance in Eighteenth-Century France.* Durham, N.C.: Duke University Press, 1946.

–––. *The Humanitarian Movement in Eighteenth-Century France.* University, Ky.: University of Kentucky Press, 1957.

McKie, Douglas. *Antoine Lavoisier: Scientist, Economist, Social Reformer.* New York: Henry Schuman, 1952.

Nickerson, Hoffman. *The Armed Horde, 1793–1939: A Study in the Rise, Survival, and Decline of the Mass Army.* New York: G. P. Putnam's Sons, 1940.

Palmer, R. R. *Twelve Who Ruled.* Princeton, N.J.: Princeton University Press, 1944.

Phipps, Ramsay Weston. *The Armies of the First French Republic and the Rise of the Marshals of Napoleon I.* Edited by C. F. Phipps and

Elizabeth Sandars. 4 vols. London: Oxford University Press, 1959.

Rieux, J., and Hassenforder, J. *Histoire de Service de Santé militaire et du Val-de-Grâce.* Paris: Charles-Lavauzelle, 1950.

Roemer, Milton I., ed. *Henry E. Sigerist on the Sociology of Medicine.* New York: MD Publications, 1960.

Rosen, George, *The Specialization of Medicine.* New York: Columbia University Press, 1944.

Rosen, George, and Caspari-Rosen, Beate. *400 Years of a Doctor's Life.* New York: Henry Schuman, 1947.

Rostand, Edmond. *Cyrano de Bergerac.* New York: Harper and Brothers, 1936.

Rudé, George, *The Crowd in the French Revolution.* Oxford: Oxford University Press, 1959.

Singer, Charles Joseph. *A Short History of Medicine.* 2d. ed. New York: Oxford University Press, 1962.

Smeaton, W. A. *Fourcroy, Chemist and Revolutionary, 1755–1809.* Cambridge, England: W. Heffer and Sons, 1962.

Soubiran, André. *Le baron Larrey, chirurgien de Napoléon.* Paris: Fayard, 1967.

Stewart, Ferdinand Campbell. *Eminent French Surgeons, With a Historical and Statistical Account of the Hospitals of Paris.* Buffalo, N.Y.: A. Burke, n.d.

Thompson, Brooks. "The Wartime Mobilization of Savants by the Committees of Public Safety." Ph.D. dissertation, University of Alabama, 1955.

Thompson, Charles J. S. *The History and Evolution of Surgical Instruments.* New York: Schuman's, 1942.

Thompson, James Matthew. *The French Revolution.* New York: Oxford University Press, 1945.

Thorwald, Jurgen. *The Century of the Surgeon.* New York: Pantheon, 1957.

Triaire, Paul. *Larrey et les campaigns de la Révolution et de l'Empire, 1768–1842.* Tours: Alfred Mame, 1902.

Turgeon, Frederick K., and Gilligan, Arthur C., eds. *The Principal Comedies of Molière.* New York: Macmillan, 1947.

Vignery, John R. "Jacobin Educational Theories and Policies in the French National Convention, 1792–94." Ph.D. dissertation, University of Wisconsin, 1960. Subsequently published as *The French Revolution and the Schools: Educational Policies of the Mountain, 1792–1794.* Madison: State Historical Society of Wisconsin, 1965.

Warner, Charles K., ed. *From the Ancien Régime to the Popular Front: Essays in the History of Modern France in Honor of Shepard B. Clough.* New York: Columbia University Press, 1969.

Weinberger, Bernhard Wolf. *Pierre Fauchard, Surgeon-Dentist; A Brief Account of the Beginning of Modern Dentistry, the First Dental Textbook, and Professional Life Two Hundred Years Ago.* Minneapolis: Pierre Fauchard Academy, 1941.

Wolf, Abraham. *A History of Science, Technology, and Philosophy in the Eighteenth Century.* 2d ed. London: George Allen and Unwin, 1952.

Yardin, A. *L'Hôpital militaire de Calais.* Paris: Imprimerie nationale, 1938.

Articles

Bonnette, P. "Rapport médicale sur la blessure du général Marceau." *Chronique médicale* 17 (1910): 78–80.

Bottet, M. "Le passé: le service de santé et les commissaires des guerres." *Caducée* 5 (1905): 151–54.

Boutry, M. "La médecine et les institutions charitables au temps de Louis XVI." *Chronique médicale* 11 (1904): 737–43.

Brienne, Maxime. "Brillat-Savarin, 'médecin-amateur'." *Chronique médicale* 28 (1921): 323–25.

"C." "Quelques évadés de la médecine et de la pharmacie: Berthollet, médecin." *Chronique médicale* 30 (1923): 99–101.

Camelin, A. "Lyon et médecine militaire." *Revue historique de l'armée* 16, no. 2 (1958): 83–94.

Cilleuls, Jean des. "Chirurgiens militaires de l'ancien régime." *Revue historique de l'armée* 6, no. 1 (1950): 7–18.

———. "Les médecins aux armées d'ancien régime." *Revue historique de l'armée* 6, no. 4 (1950): 7–24.

"Couthon, et Drouet, d'aprés les 'Souvenirs' d'Isabey." *Chronique médicale* 11 (1904): 372–73.

Da Costa, J. Chalmers. "Baron Larrey: A Sketch." *Johns Hopkins Hospital Bulletin* 17 (1906): 195–215.

Dally, J. F. Halls. "Jean Nicolas Corvisart (1755–1821), Chief Physician to Napoleon I." *Medical Record* 153 (April 2, 1941): 233–38.

"La découverte de l'anesthésie chirurgicale pour la réduction des luxations par des rebouteurs au XVIII siècle," *Archives provinciales de chirurgie* 20 (1911): 611–13.

"Le docteur-général Dessaix." *Chronique médicale* 16 (1909): 698–703.

Duveen, Denis. "Antoine Laurent Lavoisier and the French Revolution."

Journal of Chemical Education, 31: 61.

Ferron, Michel. "Le chirurgien principal de l'armée: Baron Jean Péborde, médecin du Murat (1773–1846)." *Progrès médicale* 44 (supplement illustré, 1929): 33–37.

———. "Le service de santé des armées françaises et les évacuations par eau de 1743 à 1832." *Archives de médecine et pharmacie militaire* 59 (1912): 455–71.

Fischer, George. "Surgery One Hundred Years Ago." Translated by Carl H. von Klein, *Journal of the American Medical Association* 28 (1897): 308; 29 (1897): 27; 30 (1898): 140.

Genty, Maurice, "Brillat-Savarin." *Progrès médicale* 34 (1921): 386–88.

Guillaume, M. J. "Un mot légendaire: 'La République n'a pas besoin de savants' " *La Révolution française* 38 (1900): 385.

Heizmann, Charles L. "Military Sanitation in the Sixteenth, Seventeenth, and Eighteenth Centuries." *Annals of Medical History* 1 (1917): 281–300.

Hillemand, Constant. "Histoire de la médecine." *Progrès médicale* 47, no. 40 (1932): 1658–72.

Laboulbène, J. J. A. "Histoire du journalisme médicale, 1679–1880." *Gazette des hôpitaux civils et militaires* 53, no. 137 (1880): 1057, 1065, 1073, 1088–89.

Lagnieu, Armand de. "La médecine dans Brillat-Savarin." *Progrès médicale* 36 (1923): 433–35.

Mathiez, Albert. "La mobilisation des savants en l'an II." *Revue de Paris* 24 (1917): 542–65.

———. "La mobilisation générale en l'an II." *Revue de Paris* 24 (1917): 581–602.

Paumès, M. B. "La parenté médicale du maréchal Bessières." *Chronique médicale* 20 (1913): 193–96.

Pouchet, George. "Les sciences pendant la Terreur, d'aprés les documents du temps et les pièces des Archives nationales." *La Révolution française* 30 (1896): 251–77, 333–64.

Rosen, George, "Hospitals, Medical Care and Social Policy in the French Revolution." *Bulletin of the History of Medicine* 30 (1956): 124–49.

Scott, Samuel F. "The Regeneration of the Line Army During the French Revolution." *Journal of Modern History* 42 (September, 1970): 307–30.

Temkin, Owsei. "The Role of Surgery in the Rise of Modern Medical Thought." *Bulletin of the History of Medicine* 25 (1951): 248–59.

Triaire, Paul. "Tactique sanitaire: les ambulances volantes de Larrey." *Caducée* 2 (1902): 157–59.

INDEX

*(An asterisk * denotes biographical footnote.)*